Sebastian Dinu

Gene regulation in human coronary artery endothelial cells

AF154034

Sebastian Dinu

Gene regulation in human coronary artery endothelial cells

After treatment with protein binding uremic toxins, as well as estrogen

Natural Sciences Series

Impressum / Imprint

Bibliografische Information der Deutschen Nationalbibliothek: Die Deutsche Nationalbibliothek verzeichnet diese Publikation in der Deutschen Nationalbibliografie; detaillierte bibliografische Daten sind im Internet über http://dnb.d-nb.de abrufbar.

Bibliographic information published by the Deutsche Nationalbibliothek: The Deutsche Nationalbibliothek lists this publication in the Deutsche Nationalbibliografie; detailed bibliographic data are available in the Internet at http://dnb.d-nb.de.

Coverbild / Cover image: www.ingimage.com

Verlag / Publisher:
AV Akademikerverlag
ist ein Imprint der / is a trademark of
OmniScriptum GmbH & Co. KG
Heinrich-Böcking-Str. 6-8, 66121 Saarbrücken, Deutschland / Germany
Email: info@akademikerverlag.de

Herstellung: siehe letzte Seite /
Printed at: see last page
ISBN: 978-3-639-64377-0

Table of contents

Acknowledgments

I am dedicating this book to my beloved wife, Odette Dinu, for all her caring support, encouragement and motivation throughout my studies as well as my life. She also deserves exceptional thanks for proofreading my manuscript.

A unique dedication goes to my dear children, Lucas & Sophia, who I am very proud of and who have always been a driving force during the past years. They pushed my life to a whole other level and I could not imagine it without them.

Special thanks go also to my parents, Georgeta & Cornel Dinu, for supporting and encouraging me all the way, and Graziella Dinu, for being a great sister.

Further, I would like to thank Univ.-Prof. Dr. Stylianos Kapiotis, CEO of Labcon Medizinische Laboratorien GmbH; as well as Ao. Univ.-Prof. Dipl.-Ing. Dr. Marcela Hermann, Ao. Univ.-Prof. Dr. Hilde Laggner, and Ao. Univ.-Prof. DDr. Bernhard Gmeiner, Medical University of Vienna, for making this project possible and guiding me through it.

Last but not least, I am grateful to my supervisor, Ao. Univ.-Prof. Dipl.-Ing. Dr. Florian Rüker, University of Natural Resources and Life Sciences, for the great guidance, incentive and much appreciated advice.

Preface

This work has been conducted in collaboration with Prof. Gmeiner and was financially supported by the medical and scientific fund of the mayor of the federal capital city of Vienna under the project AP10059BGM "Protein-bound uremic toxins as potential initiators of atherogenic modification of low and high density lipoproteins."

Project leader: Univ.Prof. DDr. Bernhard Gmeiner from the Vienna General Hospital and Medical University of Vienna, Institute of Medical Chemistry and Pathobiochemistry, Center of Pathobiochemistry and Genetics.

Abstract

Chronic kidney disease and cardiovascular diseases have a high prevalence in the developed countries and are also rising in emerging countries. A direct result of kidney failure is elevated protein-bound uremic toxin concentrations in the blood. While normal uremic toxins are being successfully reduced in concentration by means of standard hemodialysis, protein binding toxins accumulate in patients with chronic renal disease or kidney failure and can ultimately result in cardiovascular diseases such as atherosclerosis.

In this project, the gene expression of ten toxin treated proteins of different types (cellular adhesion molecules, enzymes, inhibitor proteins, cytokines, and receptors/cofactors) in human coronary artery endothelial cell lines was monitored by a specifically designed reverse transcription real time quantitative PCR assay using a novel, robust reference gene. Besides testing for the regulatory effect by mentioned toxins, the effect of estrogen during toxin incubation was investigated as well.

Many genes of interest show a typical reaction of toxic stimuli, while others seem to have individual behavior granting room for interpretation. Some of the typical results were up-regulation of pro-inflammatory genes such as ICAM-1, MCP-1, MMP-9, PAI-1, VCAM-1; down-regulation of eNOS, and up-regulation of Tissue Factor thus increasing risk of thrombi formation. The majority of cells incubated with estrogen showed typical cardio-protective and anti-inflammatory effects when the genes of interest were significantly toxin stimulated.

1. Introduction

1.1.   General

Cardiovascular diseases (CVDs) including coronary heart disease / coronary artery disease (CHD/CAD) are the leading cause of death in the world. The global share in cause of death is estimated at around 30 % while the percentage in Austria is estimated at over 43 % (World Health Organization, 2008).

Being a widely spread disease, year after year over 2 billion USD in research funding are distributed across the U.S. National Institutes of Health (National Institutes of Health, 2013) which results in big market opportunities for pharmaceutical companies. The FDA and EMA already approved several new drugs relating to CVDs, CHD, and CAD this year (European Medicines Agency, 2012; Food and Drug Administration, 2013).

Although there are over 100 approved pharmaceutical products on the market that target CAD alone, the best treatment is still the preventive one. Risk factors are mainly divided in varying and non-varying ones such as age, family history of CVD, sex and even race (Centers for Disease Control and Prevention, 2012; Jousilahti, Vartiainen, Tuomilehto, & Puska, 1999; Mackay, Mensah, Mendis, Greenlund, & World Health Organization., 2004). Varying factors comprise 75 % of all risk factors and are attributed to our lifestyle including habits such as indulging in an unhealthy diet, smoking, low physical activity, and alcohol abuse. These habits can result in high blood pressure, obesity, type 2 diabetes, harmful concentrations of lipids like high LDL-cholesterol or triglycerides and low HDL-cholesterol. Further risk factors worth mentioning are preceding diseases, and conditions of psychological origin such as depression, psycho-social stress and low socio-economic status (Mackay et al., 2004).

1.2. Cardiovascular and chronic kidney diseases

The CVD atherosclerosis is the leading cause of death in patients with chronic kidney disease (Sarnak et al., 2003). Progressive loss in renal function causes waste product accumulation in the bloodstream which increases the chance of a drastic CVD break out. Hemodialysis is the only way of reducing the toxin and waste concentration in the blood of a CKD patient. Unfortunately, not all of the mentioned waste products can be efficiently removed via this procedure. Some of these toxins bind very tightly to proteins like serum albumin thus creating the previously mentioned complication in dialysis (Piroddi, Bartolini, Ciffolilli, & Galli, 2013). Toxins and cellular dysfunction contribute to the calcification of arteries (Fig. 1.1) that can lead to a myocardial infarction or stroke, depending on the location. One pitfall is that atherosclerosis may develop silently without detection therefore leading to a false perception of health.

1.3. Human coronary artery endothelial cells

The general term "endothelial cells" refers to a thin layer of cells surrounding a vascular or lymphatic vessel containing the lumen. All endothelial cells in contact with blood form as monolayers the vascular *tunica intima* which is the direct barrier between the bloodstream and the surrounding tissue including the rest of the vessel. The endothelial cells that form the *tunica intima* of coronary arteries of the human *myocardium* are therefore called human coronary artery endothelial cells (HCAECs). Endothelial cells in general play a very important role in hormone trafficking as well as the selective passage of materials to or from the blood. Some endothelial cells have very distinct specializations for example cells in renal *glomeruli* that are specialized in fluid filtration. Additional common functions are angiogenesis, which is the formation of new blood vessels, the release of factors resulting in inflammation (recruitment of neutrophil granulocytes), and blood coagulation including fibrinolysis and thrombosis.

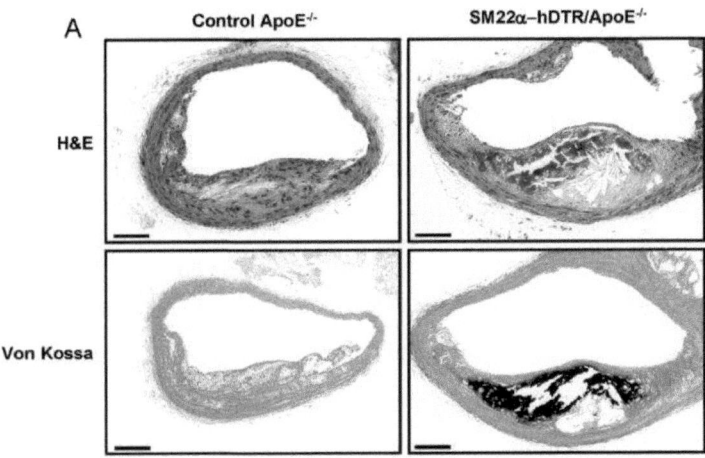

A   Control ApoE⁻/⁻   SM22α–hDTR/ApoE⁻/⁻

H&E

Von Kossa

Fig. 1.1 Progressive thickening and calcification of an artery

A hematoxylin/eosin (H&E, top) and Von Kossa (bottom) staining of brachiocephalic mouse arteries showing the area of calcification in (Apo)E$^{-/-}$ transgenic mice (left: accelerates plaques formation) and the area of calcification around the necrotic core of SM22α-hDTR/ApoE$^{-/-}$ transgenic mice (right: human diphteria toxin expression causing apoptosis, H&E: dark grey, Von Kossa: black). Figures modified after Clarke et al., 2008.

A highly significant function of HCAECs is the production of nitric oxide (NO) from L-Arginine and oxygen. When released into the bloodstream, the concentration of NO causes change in the vascular tone through vasodilatation and vasoconstriction.

Several of the analyzed protein-bound toxins show endothelial specific toxicity which causes endothelial dysfunction, leading to atherosclerosis (Jourde-Chiche, Dou, Cerini, Dignat-George, & Brunet, 2011). Since the effects of protein-bound toxins on HCAECs are not yet fully studied, it is important to understand if and which HCAEC specific gene expressions are regulated by these toxins.

1.4. The estrogen 17ß-estradiol

Estrogens are the main sexual hormones present in women. The primarily occurring estrogens estrone (E_1), estradiol (E_2) and estriol (E_3) are all androgen derived steroidal hormones. This thesis will investigate the effect of (17ß-)estradiol on the toxin-GOI expression interaction. Since the biological estradiol has a low *in vitro* stability, the synthetic analog moxestrol is used, to which a methoxylation at the 11'-C-locus and an ethinylation at the 17'-C-locus was performed (DuPont/NEN, Boston, US-MA), causing a higher stability and half-life (Hermann, Seif, Schneider, & Ivessa, 1997). In view of the fact that statistics state a lower prevalence of cardiovascular disease in pre-menopausal women than in men, some of the regulatory results of toxin treated cells should be antagonized by estrogen. Many regulatory effects of estrogens are well studied and documented, however since these hormones cause a wide variety of regulations, they still remain a key component in many field of research.

Fig. 1.2 ß-estradiol (top) and moxestrol (bottom)

1.5.   Proteins of interest

1.5.1.   Endothelial nitric oxide synthase

The endothelial nitric oxide synthase (eNOS) is part of the family of nitric oxide forming enzymes that also includes neuronal, inducible and bacterial Nitric Oxide Synthase (thus n-,i-, bNOS). It is a homodimeric enzyme of which each monomer consists of an N-terminal oxigenase domain and multiple C-terminal reductase domains. Due to its C-terminal multi-domain region, it is the only known enzyme to bind to the cofactors calmodulin, flavin adenine dinucleotide (FAD), flavin mononucleotide (FMN), heme and tetrahydrobiopterin (H_4B), which in addition to NADPH are needed for the formation of the reactive free radical nitric oxide. Unlike iNOS and nNOS, which are found in the cytosol for the most part, eNOS is the membrane associated isoenzyme found on the endothelial cell membrane as well as on the membrane of the golgi apparatus. The membrane association is due to the cotranslational N-terminal myristoylation and the post-translational palmitoylation (Liu, Hughes, & Sessa, 1997).

The production pathway of NO is a five-electron oxidation of L-arginine to L-citrulline as shown in the simplified equation below

$$2\,(L - arginine) +\ 3\,NADPH + 2\,H^+ + 4\,O_2$$
$$= 2\,(L - citrulline) + 2\,NO + 3\,NADP^+$$

while the pathway of the electrons through the cofactors can be visualized as

$$NADPH\ \rightarrow FAD \rightarrow FMN \xrightarrow{Calmodulin} heme \rightarrow NOS \qquad \text{(Roman et al., 2000)}$$

Among other location and NOS dependent functions, the NO produced by eNOS regulates through a signaling cascade the vascular tone by vasodilatation/vasoconstriction and promotes smooth muscle relaxation hence often equated with the Endothelium-derived relaxing factor (Sharma & Khanna, 2013). Further, it has been confirmed that NO functions in negative feedback regulation through reversible inhibition particularly on eNOS (Griscavage, Hobbs, & Ignarro, 1995). Although eNOS is constantly expressed from the NOS3 gene at a basal level, it has been shown that molecules like endotoxins can have a regulatory effect on the expression of eNOS (Zhou et al., 2000).

1.5.2. Intercellular adhesion molecule 1

Also known as cluster of differentiation 54 (CD54), ICAM-1 is part of the immunoglobulin superfamily. It is a transmembrane glycoprotein with one extracellular N-terminal domain facing away from the cell, the transmembrane domain and one C-terminal intracellular domain. ICAM-1 is naturally expressed at low levels on endothelial cells, leukocytes and macrophages thus playing an important role in innate immune response reactions and inflammation. The overexpression of ICAM-1 can be induced via cytokines such as interleukin-1 (IL-1) and tumor necrosis factor-α (TNF-α) not to mention also by endotoxins (Burns, Takei, & Doerschuk, 1994). It reaches its maximum concentration after ~ 24 hours which it can hold for up to 3 days (Leeuwenberg et al., 1992). When activated, the lymphocyte function-associated antigen 1 receptor (LFA-1, an integrin) from the surface of leukocytes binds to the extracellular domain of ICAM-1 and facilitates leukocyte transmigration through the endothelium to the tissue (Hopkins, Baird, & Nusrat, 2004). Some pathogens like rhinoviruses (common cold) and the parasite *Plasmodium falciparum* (Malaria) use ICAM-1 as a mediator for passing through the vascular endothelium after entering the blood stream (Chakravorty & Craig, 2005; Greve et al., 1989).

1.5.3. Monocyte chemotactic protein 1

MCP-1 is a small cytokine also known as chemokine C-C motif ligand 2 (CCL2) that acts as a recruiter of various cells of the immune system. It is anchored on the outside of endothelial cells via glycosaminoglycan side chains of proteoglycans hence being in direct contact with the blood. The intracellular MCP-1 signaling is mediated by the G-protein linked C-C chemokine receptors 2 & 4 (CCR2 & 4). The expression level varies depending on various factors. The activation occurs by cleavage of the MCP-1 proprotein through matrix metalloprotease 12 (MMP-12) whereupon it attracts dendritic cells, monocytes and T cells to sites of inflammation and/or infection which in their turn also secrete MCP-1 to start an attractive as to facilitate the recruitment of more cells (Carr, Roth, Luther, Rose, & Springer, 1994). Since atherosclerosis also causes inflammation of the thickened arterial site, MCP-1 plays a major role in involuntarily "luring" the cells to the inflamed site where it, together with LDL-cholesterol and other plaque-forming materials, contributes to calcifying the artery.

1.5.4.   Matrix metalloprotease 2 & 9

Matrix metalloproteases are enzymes responsible for the breakdown of extracellular matrix for example in embryonic development, tissue remodeling and disease processes.

MMP-2 & -9 both proteolytically digest type IV collagens. Since this type of collagen is mainly found in the basal lamina of cell membranes, both enzymes play an important role in facilitating the disintegration of the matrix.

MMP-2 has been shown to have an important role in the regulation of angiogenesis and response to inflammation, while MMP-9 has been identified as a potential biological marker for the development of some carcinomas (Colovic et al., 2013).

1.5.5.   Plasminogen activator inhibitor 1

Due to the fact that PAI-2 is produced in the placenta and hence only at significant levels during pregnancy, this paragraph will introduce the main representative of the four PAI proteins, PAI-1. PAIs are proteins that inhibit the activity of serine proteases, thus also the name serpins. Therefore they regulate the activity of enzyme activating proteases by lock-and-key competitive inhibition at the active site (Egelund et al., 1998). PAI-1 is primarily produced by the liver and vascular endothelial cells but since it plays a crucial role in blood clot lysis, the vast majority of it is found in thrombocytes. Plasminogen activator proteins like tissue plasminogen activator (tPA) and urokinase-type plasminogen activator (uPA) are responsible for the activity of plasmin, a serine protease regulating fibrinolysis. Both, tPA and uPA are controlled via inhibition through PAI-1. The visualization in Fig. 1.3 shows the pathway of the PAI-1 mediated activation. But it should be mentioned that a number of activators and inhibitors as well as other enzymes such as the coagulation factor XII and kallikreins can proteolytically activate plasmin. Remarkably, when PAI-1 releases the plasminogen activator from its inhibition, the precursor protein plasminogen is proteolytically cleaved by t-/u-PA to the active serine protease plasmin (Castellino & Ploplis, 2005).

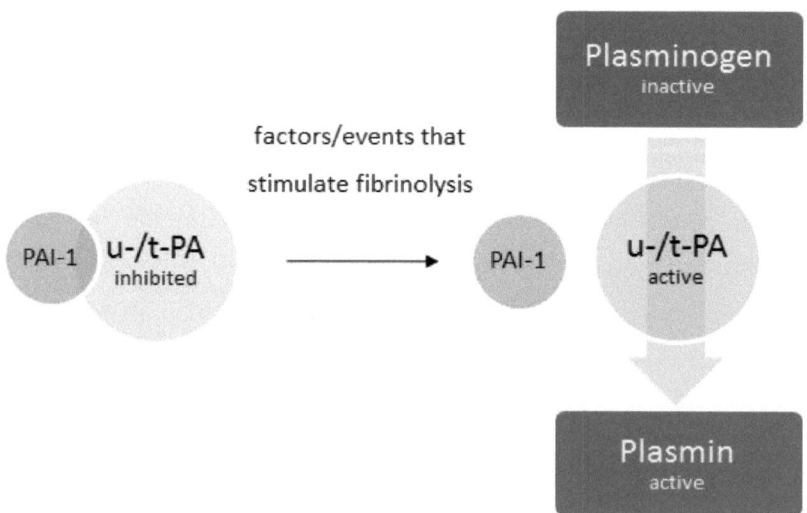

Fig. 1.3 Role of PAI-1 in plasminogen/plasmin activation

Although events such as unwanted blood clotting trigger the release of PAI-1 from PA, other stimuli such as TNF-α, TGF-β positively regulate the expression of PAI-1. It is also well documented that PAI-1 levels are elevated in the elderly and that conditions such as obesity, emotional stress, and vascular sclerosis cause an up-regulation (Yamamoto, Takeshita, Kojima, Takamatsu, & Saito, 2005), not to mention *in vitro* co-cultivation of endothelial cells with smooth muscle cells (Gallicchio et al., 1994).

In the active state, plasmin is able to digest a variety of blood plasma proteins but mainly fibrin. Since the matured fibrin mesh is a matrix of many polymerized fibrin monomers, the result of the plasmin digestion are many fragments with a wide range in molecular weight (Fig. 1.4). The fibrinolytic reaction is also controlled by a variety of factors for example at the plasminogen → plasmin step through inhibitors such as $α_2$-antiplasmin and $α_2$-macroglobulin.

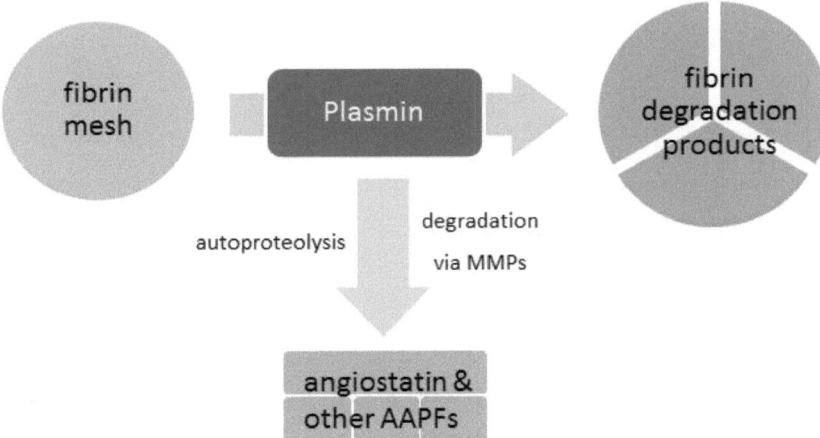

Fig. 1.4 Fibrin and plasmin degradation

The horizontal arrow visualizes the fibrin mesh breakdown by plasmin, while the vertical arrow visualizes the plasmin degradation

A further, non-reversible step is the degradation of plasmin either through autoproteolysis or enzymatically by proteases like elastase and various matrix metalloproteases (Waisman, 2003). The products of this degradation are anti-angiogenic plasminogen fragments (AAPFs) including angiostatin, which has been well studied and is researched for the use in cancer therapy as a growth blocker.

1.5.6.　E-selectin

Selectins are part of one of the four Ig-like superfamilies and are essentially cell adhesion molecules. To this date, three types of selectins are characterized: E-selectin, which is solely found on the surface of (stimulated) endothelial cells; L-selectin, which is found on lymphocytes; and P-selectin, which is found on stimulated endothelial cells and stimulated platelets. The difference between E- and P-selectin is not only the additional expression of P-selectin on platelets, but also the difference in availability. E-selectin is (significantly) expressed and secreted directly to the surface after stimulation of endothelial cells with cytokines, endotoxins, TNF-α and IL-1 with a maximum after 6-12 hours ensuing a decline to the baseline after ~ 24 hours (Leeuwenberg et al., 1992). P-selectin on the other hand, can be stored in endothelial Weibel-Palade bodies and thrombocytic α-granules of inactive endothelial cells and thrombocytes (Wagner, 1993).

1.5.7.　Thrombomodulin

Thrombomodulin is an integral membrane protein involved in the regulation of blood coagulation by acting as a cofactor to thrombin. Its extracellular domain modulates the conversion of thrombin from a procoagulant to an anticoagulant enzyme thus converting indirectly activated protein Ca from the precursor protein C. Finally, protein Ca reduces the amount of functional thrombin by cleaving activated cofactors (V and VIII) of the coagulation system. Thrombomodulin is mainly found on endothelial cells but is also expressed on monocytes, some dentritic cells and mesothelial cells (Verhagen et al., 1996).

1.5.8. Tissue factor

While Thrombomodulin reduces blood coagulation, Tissue Factor enables it. Triggered by a trauma such as tissue damage, the cryptic protein becomes coagulantly active and the extracellular domain of this (mainly) transmembrane protein activates in combination with factor VIIa the coagulation factor X. The now activated factor Xa activates the procoagulant protein thrombin with the help of factor Va. The burst of thrombin in the bloodstream results in a fast thrombus formation crucial to thrombosis (V. M. Chen, 2013). Located mainly on subendothelial tissue cells, it is primarily cut off from the bloodstream however, when injury occurs, the above mentioned cascade is activated (Konigsberg, Kirchhofer, Riederer, & Nemerson, 2001). Two alternatively spliced products exist: the membrane-bound and the soluble form. The latter lacks exon 5, thus exon 4 is directly spliced to exon 6. Since the studied object in this thesis is the HCAEC, the primers for Tissue Factor in 3.1 where designed spanning the exon junction 5-6 hence resulting in no amplification of soluble Tissue Factor.

1.5.9. Vascular cell adhesion molecule 1

Like other cell adhesion molecules, VCAM-1 is part of the immunoglobulin superfamily with 6-7 Ig-like domains. VCAM-1 is strongly expressed on endothelial cells after stimulation with cytokines like TNF-α and IL-1 and facilitates the aggregation of macrophages and other white blood cells to inflammatory sites. Therefore it not only is involved in atherosclerosis and rheumatoid arthritis but it also has been well studied that tumor cells exploit CAMs like VCAM-1 to pass the vascular barrier and infiltrate further tissue (Q. Chen, Zhang, & Massague, 2011).

1.6.   Uremic protein-bound toxins

The following will grant some insight into the toxins studied. All of the toxins examined are either polyamines or organic compounds with aromatic groups. Seeing as how these toxins are also found in healthy individuals, the concentration that is co-regulated by the kidneys is of utmost importance. In the case of renal failure, the resulting waste accumulation also increases the toxicity of those small molecular compounds. The fact that normal hemodialysis is very inefficient in removing them calls for new techniques in lowering their presence either through high-efficiency protein-leaking dialyzers, frequent/daily dialysis, adsorption techniques or pharmacological therapy that lowers the formation rate of the toxins or causes dissociation from the proteins and hence facilitates standard hemodialysis (Piroddi et al., 2013). All structure figures were taken from Chemspider (Royal Society of Chemistry).

1.6.1.   Cadaverine

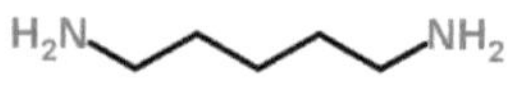

Cadaverine belongs to the alkanamine family and is also known under the IUPAC name 1,5-pentane-1,5-diamine. It is a foul-smelling polyamine produced by

H_2N ⌁ NH_2

Fig. 1.5 Cadaverine

protein hydrolysis during putrefaction of animal tissue but in living beings, it is formed by intestinal bacterial decarboxylation of lysine through lysine decarboxylase. Interestingly, it is detected even in the central nervous system wherefrom the highest concentration was measured in the brain during hibernation (Dolezalova, Stepita-Klauco, & Fairweather, 1974). It shows acute toxicity when ingested, inhaled or absorbed by skin (National Institutes of Health & National Library of Medicines, 2011) and like other polyamines, is involved in the cellular proliferation regulation.

1.6.2. p-cresol

p-cresol is an aromatic organic compound derived from phenol known under the IUPAC name 4-methylphenol. It is produced during nutritional protein breakdown and excreted with urine. Therefore, renal dysfunction causes p-cresol accumulation in the bloodstream. Besides being toxic,

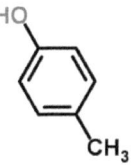

Fig. 1.6 p-cresol

irritating and carcinogenic, it has been shown to tightly bind to solubilized proteins causing increased amounts of free p-cresol and simultaneously hypoalbuminemia (De Smet et al., 2003). Furthermore, phagocyte function is being inhibited and the adhesion ability of leukocytes to cytokine stimulated endothelial cells is being reduced, hence facilitating pathogenic infection (Brunet, Dou, Cerini, & Berland, 2003).

1.6.3. Hippuric acid

This compound is a carboxylic acid formed from benzoic acid and glycine, thus the trivial name N-benzoylglycine. Furthermore, it is formed after being exposed to aromatic compounds such as toluene or benzol over benzoic acid to hippuric

Fig. 1.7 Hippuric acid

acid, to then be excreted through the urinary system (Pero, 2010). A further source of educts for hippuric acid formation is plant based foodstuff containing quinic acid. Research has also shown, that hippuric acid is highly toxic for microbial pathogens hence the beneficial moderately elevated levels in urine during a bacterial urinary tract infection (Raz, Chazan, & Dan, 2004). Other research has shown, that high concentrations of hippuric acid have an inhibitory effect on glucose exploitation in the muscle, as well as a high serum concentration is also correlated with neurological symptoms of uremia (Brunet et al., 2003).

1.6.4.   Indoxyl sulfate

Indoxyl sulfate is an aryl sulfate produced as a secondary metabolite from dietary protein breakdown (The European Bioinformatics Institute, 2012). It is a circulating uremic toxin that has been proven to accelerate the progression of renal failure by inducing

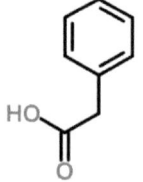

Fig. 1.8 Indoxyl sulfate

glomerular sclerosis and interstitial fibrosis (Aoyama, Miyazaki, & Niwa, 1999; Brunet et al., 2003). Further negative effects of indoxyl sulfate are the induction of free radicals in smooth muscle cells and vascular endothelial cells as well as the reduced production of nitric oxide in endothelial cells by inhibition of nitric oxide synthase. In addition, it elevates the senescence of cells and promotes aortic calcification and aortic wall thickening in combination with hypertonia. Regarding these highly negative effects of indoxyl sulfate, the significantly elevated levels of this nephro-vascular toxin in the blood system is very detrimental (Niwa, 2010; Niwa & Shimizu, 2012).

1.6.5.   Phenylacetic acid

This carboxylic acid occurs in fact naturally in plants as an auxin and secondary metabolite. In humans, it is either produced by oxidation from phenethylamine by monoamine oxidase, intestinal bacteria such as the *Group IV Clostridium botulinum* (Collins & East, 1998) or simply by exposure to environmental phenylacetic acid. At increased levels such

Fig. 1.9 Phenyl-acetic acid

as in patients with end-stage kidney dysfunction, it inhibits the expression of inducible nitric oxide synthase (iNOS) which indirectly lowers the nitric oxide concentration in the blood. Since nitric oxide has a preventive effect against inflammation, this inhibition most likely contributes to increased atherosclerosis (Jankowski et al., 2003). Previously, it has also been determined that phenylacetic acid noncompetitively inhibits the plasma membrane bound Ca^{2+} ATPase of patients with chronic kidney disease thus resulting in pathological Ca^{2+} accumulation within tissues. This kind of accumulation may be associated with cerebral symptoms of uremia as well as derangement of the parathyroid hormone metabolism (Arieff & Massry, 1974; Jankowski et al., 1998).

1.6.6. Putrescine

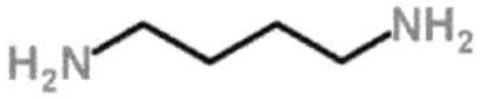

Putrescine is a polyamine like cadaverine except with butane as the base alkane (Butane-1,4-diamine). Its effects, toxicity and origin are also similar to

Fig. 1.10 Putrescine

cadaverine including the fouling smell. Furthermore, polyamines such as putrescine, spermidine and spermine are shown to inhibit erythropoietin and reduce erythropoiesis at concentrations found in patients with renal failure. Subsequently, the lower erythropoietin concentration leads to pathogenic renal anemia (Yoshida et al., 2006).

1.6.7. Spermidine

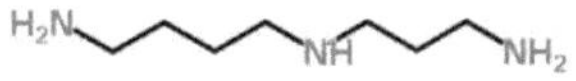

This is a polyamine with a significantly higher molecular weight than cadaverine and putrescine. It contains three aminyl groups and is synthesized

Fig. 1.11 Spermidine

from putrescine via spermidine synthase that uses S-adenosylmethioninamine (SAM) as the propylamine donor. Like putrescine, it negatively affects erythropoiesis but also inhibits neuronal nitric oxide Synthase (Hu, Mahmoud, & el-Fakahany, 1994). The latter could be caused by the fact that putrescine, spermidine and spermine share some basic structural features with L-arginine, which is an oxidation substrate of nitric oxide synthase. Therefore, as opposed to the noncompetitive inhibition of erythropoietin, the inhibitory mechanism applied here is competitive. The rank in order of decreasing K_i and therefore increasing inhibition potency is putrescine < spermidine < spermine.

1.6.8. Spermine

Transferring another propylamine group from SAM to spermidine by spermine synthase produces spermine. While it also

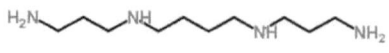

Fig. 1.12 Spermine

is responsible for cellular metabolism, similar to the precursor molecules it inhibits erythropoietin and nitric oxide synthase. From the mentioned polyamines cadaverine, putrescine, spermidine and spermine, the toxicity increases in the order of the molecular weight (Til, Falke, Prinsen, & Willems, 1997).

2. Aim of the project

The objective of this work is divided into two experimental parts. In experiment one, the affects of the toxin cocktail, consisting of all toxins from 1.6 with each having a concentration of 100 mM, are studied on the genes of interest from 1.5. It is known that certain environmental substances (e.g. endotoxins of gram-negative bacteria, TNF-α) cause a strong gene regulation for certain genes. Considering the previous facts and the symptoms patients experience, it is expected that the toxin cocktail should also trigger some regulation in gene expression.

As already mentioned in 1.1, patient gender plays an important role in the level of risk for cardiovascular diseases. Studies show, that due to a significantly higher estrogen concentration, premenopausal women are less prone to succumb to cardiovascular diseases (Jousilahti et al., 1999). Therefore, in experiment two, the influence of moxestrol (synthetic 17β-estradiol/E_2 analog) in physiological concentration on the cells is studied, and the data is compared to experiment one.

The combined aim is to detect gene regulation caused by the toxins and/or estrogen.

3. Materials and Methods

3.1. Assay validation

3.1.1. Primer design

The primers for the genes of interest (GOI) and the potential references genes (RG) were designed using NCBI's Primer-BLAST tool. Firstly, the appropriate NCBI NM accession numbers were queried to be used as templates for Primer-BLAST (Tab. 3.1). The settings for the primer jobs were set to span exon-exon junctions to avoid genomic DNA amplification. Furthermore, the melting temperatures were set to reach an optimal PCR annealing temperature of 60°C ± 3°C later on. Since the primers of the reverse transcription step are $(dT)_{18}$ oligonucleotides, the designed PCR primers had to be complementary to a region as close as possible to the 3' end and therefore the polyA-tail of the gene. This is done to minimize the errors caused by inefficient elongation caused by the reverse transcriptase. The primers were also designed to produce amplicon sizes of 70 – 200 bp (exceptionally up to 270 bp). To estimate the thermodynamic probability of hairpin and homo-/hetero dimeric formation, the selected primers were benchmarked using the OligoAnalyzer 3.1 tool (Integrated DNA Technologies Inc., Coralville, US-IA). Ultimately, the primers were ordered at Biomers.net GmbH (Ulm, DE).

Tab. 3.1 Primer overview

gene	NCBI Accession #	fwd primer	rev primer
ß2M	NM_004048.2	agatgagtatgcctgccgtg	tcatccaatccaaatgcggc
G6PDH	NM_000402.3	aaacggtcgtacacttcggg	tccgactgatggaaggcatc
GAPDH	NM_002046.4	gtcagccgcatcttcttttgc	agttaaaagcagccctggtga
HUWE1	NM_031407.5	aggttcctccggtttaggct	ccatgggtgattcctccctc
POLR2A	NM_000937.4	gaggagtttcggctcagtgg	tggcagacacaccagcatag
RPL37A	NM_000998.4	gatctggcactgtggttcct	gatggcggactttaccgtga
eNOS	NM_000603.4	atcccccggagaatggagag	agtgggtctgagcaggagat
ICAM-1	NM_000201.2	tgatgggcagtcaacagctaa	ggcagcgtagggtaaggtt
MCP-1	NM_002982.3	gcagccaccttcattcccca	cacagatctccttggccacaat
MMP-2	NM_004530.4	tgatggcatcgctcagatcc	ggcctcgtataccgcatcaa
MMP-9	NM_004994.2	acgacgtcttccagtaccga	ctggttcaactcactccggg
PAI-1	NM_000602.4	cacaaatcagacggcagcac	gagctgggcactcagaatgt
SelE	NM_000450.2	gactttctgctgctggactct	tagtaggcaagaagggccaga
TF	NM_001993.4	gagtacagacagcccggtag	agtagctccaacagtgcttcc
THBD	NM_000361.2	acatcctggacgacggtttc	cgcagatgcactcgaaggta
VCAM-1	NM_001078.3	aattccacgctgaccctgag	ggccaccactcatctcgatt

3.1.2. Cell preparation

The cryopreserved HCAECs (cat. no. C-12221) were provided by PromoCell GmbH (Heidelberg, DE), cultivated in Endothelial Cell Growth Medium MV (PromoCell), and passaged according to standard cell culture procedures. Only passages between 5 and 10 were used for the following experiments. The growth conditions were kept constant at 37°C and 5% CO_2 throughout the experiments. To assess the molecular biological conditions in the subsequent experiments, cells were seeded into two 75 cm² flasks. After reaching ~80% confluence, cells from one flask were incubated for 18 hours only in HBSS medium containing 100 µg/l HSA (Sigma-Aldrich), and served as the control cells. The other cells where incubated in HBSS/HSA medium also containing the toxin cocktail (Tab. 3.2) of 100 mM each. All toxins, the HBSS medium and HSA were provided by Sigma-Aldrich Corp. and its subsidiaries (St. Louis, US-MO).

Tab. 3.2 Toxins in their commercial form

Substance
Cadaverine.2HCl
p-Cresol
Hippuric acid 98%
(Potassium-) Indoxyl sulfate
Phenylacetic acid
Putrescine.2HCl
Spermidin.3HCl
Spermine.4HCl

Afterwards, the cells where harvested and centrifuged at 500 *rcf* for 3 mins, the resulting pellet which was used for the RNA isolation process, was purified based on silica membrane spin column technology using the GeneJET RNA Purification Kit (Thermo Fisher Scientific, Waltham, US-MA). The isolation of total RNA was conducted according to protocol which consists of cell lysis with a lysis buffer containing 40 mM dithiotreitol (DTT) and several washing steps with two different washing buffers, both containing ethanol. The elution was performed in 100 µl nuclease-free molecular grade water, which was provided with the kit. Subsequently, the RNA concentration was assessed in optical duplicates (Tab. 3.3) by means of the NanoDrop 2000 UV/VIS Spectrophotometer (Thermo Fisher).

Tab. 3.3 Total RNA concentration

sample	conc. [ng/µl]	A_{260}/A_{280}
control cells (C)	115	1,95
treated cells (T)	46	1,87

All steps involving enzymes and/or nucleic acid solutions where conducted on a 0°C cooling block.

Prior to further handling, the RNA-concentration of (C) was diluted 2,5 fold with DEPC-water to result in an RNA concentration of ~ 46 ng/µl. Since assay performance is also influenced by template concentration and not merely physical parameters, this dilution step was performed proceeding further experiments rather than between reverse transcription (RT) and PCR/Real-

Time PCR (qPCR). The successive steps were performed in triplicates (Ca,b,c; Ta,b,c) to evaluate the intra-assay variance.

3.1.3. Digestion of genomic DNA and Reverse Transcription

To assess the necessity of gDNA removal from the experiments, the six reaction samples underwent DNase I digestion in presence of 10 mM $MnCl_2$ (Tab. 3.4). In presence of Mn^{2+} ions, DNase I randomly cleaves both DNA strands resulting in blunt or sticky ends with very short overhangs (Fig. 3.1, top). Therefore the use of Mn^{2+} ions were preferred over Mg^{2+} ions, which only causes the DNase to cleave each DNA strand independently and randomly (Fig. 3.1, bottom) thus not fragmenting the DNA.

Tab. 3.4 Reaction set-up for gDNA digestion per assay

reagent		volume
Eluate, total RNA		20 µl = 920 ng
10X reaction buffer		3 µl
$MnCl_2$ 100 mM		3 µl
RiboLock	1 u/µl	1 µl
DNase I	1 u/µl	1 µl
DEPC-H_2O		2 µl
Total		30 µl

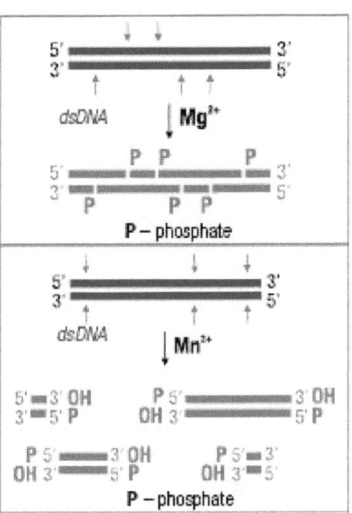

Fig. 3.1 Comparison between DNase I activity in presence of Mg^{2+} (top) and Mn^{2+} ions (bottom) (Thermo Fisher Scientific Inc., 2013)

The assays were incubated on a heat block for 30 minutes at 37 ℃. Since heating up RNA in presence of bivalent ions has a RNA-degrading effect, prior to the DNase inactivation step, 9 µl 50 mM EDTA were added. The DNase I inactivation was performed for 10 minutes at 65 ℃. Due to compulsory template dilution, the con centration is estimated at 24 ng/µl in a volume of 39 µl/sample.

Subsequently, the whole solution was used for reverse transcription. For easier dispensing and less pipetting variability, two premixes where created. The sample premix (Tab. 3.5a), which consisted of primers and nucleotides, and the enzyme premix (Tab. 3.5b), which consisted of the enzymes and buffer. After the sample solutions were added to the pre-dispensed sample premix, the enzyme premix was added and the solution was mixed by up and down suction with the pipette and then subsequently spun down.

Tab. 3.5a Sample premix composition per assay

reagent	volume
Oligo (dT) primer 100 µM	4 µl
dNTP Mix, 10 mM each	4 µl
DEPC-Water	11 µl
Total	19 µl

Tab. 3.5b Enzyme premix composition per assay

reagent	volume
5x RT buffer	16 µl
RiboLock 40 u/µl	2 µl
Rev. Transcriptase 200 u/µl	4 µl
Total	22 µl

The incubation was performed thereafter for 30 minutes at 50 ℃ followed by an inactivation step at 85 ℃ for 5 minutes. The to tal end volume was 80 µl/sample with a total initial template concentration of approximately 11,5 ng/µl.

3.1.4.   Determination of optimal PCR conditions

As stated in 3.1.1., the primers were designed to have an annealing temperature of ~ 60 ℃. To check the optimal anneal ing temperature, gradient PCR experiments using the Multigene Gradient thermal cycler (Labnet Inc., Edison, US-NJ) were conducted. An automated gel electrophoresis on the ScreenTape DS12 running on the 2200 TapeStation (both Agilent

Technologies Inc., Santa Clara, US-CA) was also performed. Given that all primers were designed to have a similar melting temperature, the range test for the annealing temperature using MyTaq DNA Polymerase (Bioline Reagents Ltd., London, UK) was firstly performed with primers for *Glyceraldehyde 3-phosphate dehydrogenase (GAPDH)* and *ß$_2$-microglobulin* (B2M). The thermocycler was programmed to have a gradient T_a consisting of $53,9 - 56,3 - 57,8 - 60 - 61,9 - 64,3$ ℃ (Tab. 5b). The reaction concentration of the primers was chosen to be 200 nM each (Tab. 3.6a). After diluting the cDNA solution 10 fold, 2 µl were used as template.

Tab. 3.6a PCR reaction set-up

reagent	volume
5x Buffer	10 µl
fwd primer	1 µl
rev primer	1 µl
Polymerase 5 u/µl	0,5 µl
ddH$_2$O	35,5 µl
Total	48 µl

Tab. 3.6b PCR cycling conditions

cycles	temperature	time
1	95℃	2'
30	95℃	15"
	53,9-64,3℃	15"
	72℃	10"
1	72℃	10'

After narrowing down the optimal annealing temperature range, the gradient PCR assay was repeated including primers of all GOIs and RGs and the gradient T_a was set to $58 - 59,9 - 62,3$ ℃.

3.1.5. Reference gene selection

Since the RNA source of this research project is the endothelial cell, the use of one robust reference gene suffices. As a result, all potential reference genes with specific amplification tested in 3.1.4 were also benchmarked via a real-time PCR (Tab. 3.7b) with a consecutive standard melting-curve analysis ranging from 60 to 90 ℃. All samples (3x C & 3x T) were therefore processed as individual samples and 1 µl per sample was used as template at all times. Using only the primers for the reference genes, that passed the specificity testing in 3.1.4, the amplification was performed with the Maxima SYBR Green 2x qPCR Master Mix (Thermo Scientific) on the ABI 7500 Real-Time

PCR System (Life Technologies Inc., Carlsbad, US-CA). Since qPCR offers a variety of detection methods, due to economical reasons, a ready to use qPCR Kit containing SYBR Green I was chosen.

Tab. 3.7a Real Time PCR reaction set-up

reagent	volume
2x qPCR Master Mix	12,5 µl
fwd primer	0,75 µl
rev primer	0,75 µl
ddH$_2$O	10 µl
Total	24 µl

Tab. 3.7b Real Time PCR cycling conditions

cycles	temperature	time
1	95℃	10'
40	95℃	15"
	60℃	30"
	72℃	32"*

*) Instrument & assay dependent variation of the reading time (31-33"), given by the software

The resulting amplification and melting curves were examined visually and the cycle of threshold (Ct) values were subjected to statistical analysis using Medcalc (MedCalc Software bvba, Ostend, BE) and Microsoft Excel.

3.1.6.   Relative primer efficiency

Although all chosen primers performed well, some did better than others. Hence the best and the two worst performing where benchmarked against the selected reference gene. Consequently, qPCR assays containing five different amounts of template (48 – 24 – 4,8 – 2,4 –0,48 ng) were performed. Their ΔC_t relative to the RG was plotted against the template amount and their slope was calculated. A slope of 0 represents identical primer efficiencies between tested GOI and RG. Slopes between -0,1 and 0,1 are acceptable.

3.2. Experiments

The cell preparation was conducted similar to 3.1.2 with the exception of the toxin treated cells. To track eventual gene regulatory trends, the four flasks had different incubation times (2 - 4 - 6 - 24 hours). After each individual incubation step, the cells were harvested and stored at − 80℃ until all samples were ready to undergo the RNA isolation process resulting in 100 µl eluate per sample. The total RNA concentration was again measured using the NanoDrop 2000. Further, the investigation of gDNA traces in the pre-RT eluate showed no amplification of gDNA except for Thrombomodulin, which has only one exon. The experiment determined the ratio of gDNA/mRNA template impurity for Thrombomodulin to be at 1:1.000 or 0,1 %. Since the gDNA digestion assays diluted the template drastically and caused great variation, in agreement with the supervisors, the impurity was considered insignificant and acceptable; therefore the experiments were conducted without removal of gDNA. The experiments were numbered as 1 (without E_2 incubation) and 2 (with E_2 incubation).

3.2.1. Experiment 1

Cell preparation and reverse transcription

Cells were cultivated, treated and harvested analogously to 3.1.2 except with incubation times of both controls and toxin treated cells of 2 - 4 - 6 - 24 hours. RNA isolation was performed as described in 3.1.2 resulting in 100 µl RNA-solution/sample of which the concentration was determined using the NanoDrop. Tab. 3.8 shows concentration and quality of the eluates.

Tab. 3.8 Total RNA concentration

sample	conc. [ng/µl]	A_{260}/A_{280}
K2	572	2,01
K4	707	2,06
K6	911	2,01
K24	131	1,96
T2	513	1,99
T4	351	2,01
T6	462	2,01
T24	192	2,04

Subsequently, the samples were prepared for reverse transcription. A special sample premix was mixed for each sample (Tab. 3.9a) which was afterwards divided into triplicates for intra-assay variation assessment. During this step, the concentrations were also adjusted to a similar level. One premix was for three reactions/sample thus creating triplicates. Since the enzyme composition is the same for all, one master mix (Tab. 3.9b) was made for all samples.

Tab. 3.9a Sample premix per sample

reagent	vol. [µl]	dilution of samples [µl RNA + µl DEPC-H$_2$O]					
		K0,K24	K2,T2,T6	K4	K6	T4	T24
Eluate, diluted	50	50 + 0	12 + 38	9 + 41	7 + 43	18 + 32	32 + 18
Oligo(dT)-Primer 100 µM	4						
dNTP Mix 10 mM each	4						
Total	58						
Total/reaction (~1,4-1,7 µg RNA)	14,5						

Tab. 3.9b Enzyme mix per reaction

reagent	vol. [µl]
5x RT Buffer	4
RiboLock 40 u/µl	0,5
RT 200 u/µl	1
Total	5,5

After preparing the mixtures, 14,5 µl from each sample premix was taken and divided into three reactions (replicate a-c). 5,5 µl enzyme mix was then added to it. Subsequent up and down suction with a pipette insured careful homogenization of the reagents. The incubation was performed at 50℃ for 30 minutes with a final inactivation step of 85℃ for 5 minutes.

Real Time PCR and data analysis

As determined in 3.1 and suggested by the manufacturer of the qPCR reagents, 1 µl of the cDNA solution was used as template. To minimize pipetting variation that comes with repetitive handling of small liquid volumes, the water and template volumes for the qPCR master mix described in 3.1.5 were adjusted. Each gene from each sample has to be relatively quantified hence resulting in a great source of handling error and therefore data variation. To avoid such complications, the cDNA solution was diluted 10-fold resulting in a greater handling volume. Hence, the water ratio in the master mix was reduced (Tab. 3.10).

Tab. 3.10a Real Time PCR reaction set-up

reagent	volume
2x qPCR Master Mix	12,5 µl
fwd primer	0,50 µl
rev primer	0,50 µl
ddH$_2$O	1,50 µl
Total	15 µl

Tab. 3.10b Real Time PCR cycling conditions

cycles	temperature	time
1	95℃	10'
40	95℃	15"
	60℃	30"
	72℃	32"*

*) 31-33", given by the software, see Tab. 3.6b in 3.5.1

A separate master mix was created and pre-dispensed for each gene into a 96-well PCR plate to which 10 µl diluted cDNA template was added and mixed by up and down suction, thus creating a sample vs. gene matrix as exemplified in Tab. 3.11. Succeeding the qPCR run, standard melting curve analysis was performed ranging from 60℃ - 90℃.

Tab. 3.11 Example of a qPCR plate sample matrix

RPL37A	eNOS	ICAM-1	MCP-1	MMP-2	MMP-9	PAI-1	SelE	TF	TM	VCAM-1
K#a										
K#b										
K#c										
T#a										
T#b										
T#c										
ntc										

Raw data analysis was performed using the system's SDS Software (v. 1.4). While the baselines were set to be chosen automatically according to the curves' kinetics, the thresholds were set manually to the beginning of the exponential phase of the amplification curve. The calculated values (Ct, Tm) where exported as *"comma separated value"* text files (.csv) and imported in Microsoft Excel.

The analysis of the Ct-values was performed using Microsoft Excel, implementing the $2^{-\Delta\Delta Ct}$ method (Livak & Schmittgen, 2001). This method was chosen due to its accurate calculation taking into account biological variation. Seeing how it requires a reference gene as well as an untreated control, the reference gene in this experiment (RG, called calibrator in the above publication) is RPL37A. The control is the extract of the untreated cells of the given incubation time.

$$\Delta\Delta C_t = (C_{t,GOI} - C_{t,RG})_{treated} - (C_{t,GOI} - C_{t,RG})_{control}$$

The fold change is being calculated by putting 2 to the power of the negative $\Delta\Delta C_t$, as previously mentioned. In case $2^{-\Delta\Delta Ct}$ is below 1, the negative fold change is calculated as $-\frac{1}{2^{-\Delta\Delta Ct}}$. This transformation is necessary to avoid fold changes between -1 and 1. By definition, a fold change of 1 means no change while >1 represents up-regulation and <-1 represents down-regulation. Values between -1 and 1 are therefore not permitted. For fold change visualization, the values have been corrected to have 0 as the reference point (e.g. -1,8 → -0,8; 2,3 → 1,3) and plotted against the toxin incubation time.

3.2.2.   Experiment 2

This experiment differs from the previous one by studying the influence of estrogen on the toxin - GOI interaction. Cell preparation was conducted similar to experiment 1 with the exception of a 24 h pre-incubation and continuous incubation with 50 nM moxestrol during toxin treatment.

Tab. 3.12 Total RNA concentration

sample	conc. [ng/µl]	A_{260}/A_{280}
KE2	970	2,00
KE4	680	2,05
KE6	460	2,01
KE24	300	2,00
TE2	550	2,08
TE4	555	2,05
TE6	320	2,00
TE24	350	2,07

Subsequently, the samples were prepared for reverse transcription as in experiment 1.

Tab. 3.13a Sample premix per sample

reagent	vol. [µl]	dilution of samples [µl RNA + µl DEPC-H_2O]				
		KE2	KE4	KE6	KE24, TE6, TE24	TE2, TE4
Eluate, diluted	50	6,4 + 43,6	8,8 + 41,2	14+36	20+30	12+38
Oligo(dT)-Primer 100 µM	4					
dNTP Mix 10 mM each	4					
Total	58					
Total/reaction (~1,4-1,7 µg RNA)	14,5					

Tab. 3.13b Enzyme mix per reaction

reagent	vol. [µl]
5x RT Buffer	4
RiboLock 40 u/µl	0,5
RT 200 u/µl	1
Total	5,5

The mixtures were again divided into three reactions (replicate a-c) and 5,5 µl enzyme mix was added to each reaction setup. After mixing, the incubation was performed at 50°C for 30 minutes with a final i nactivation step of 85°C for 5 minutes.

Subsequently, the 10 fold dilution, qPCR and raw data analysis was performed exactly as in experiment 1.

4. Results & Discussion

4.1.   Assay validation

4.1.1.   Reference gene

The mentioned reference gene candidates were recommended by numerous publications as more stable alternatives to traditional reference genes such as GAPDH, which can have a high variability (Maltseva et al., 2013). As shown in Tab. 4.1, from all RGs only ß2M, GAPDH and RPL37A resulted in specific amplification, with minor primer dimer formation from the GAPDH oligonucleotides.

Tab. 4.1 Overview over the specificity of the reference gene candidate primers

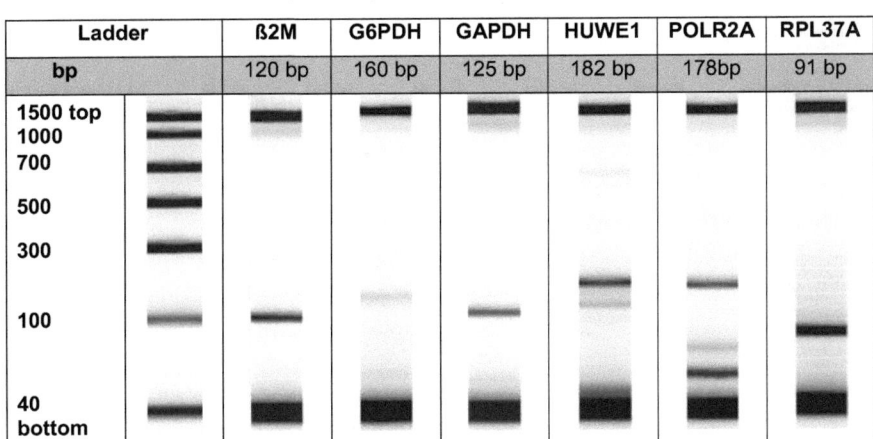

The qPCR application of these three candidates resulted in smooth amplification curves with the exception of an apparent technical inhibition of exactly the same replicate in ß2M and GAPDH. Nevertheless, magnification of the region of threshold results in a preliminary visual graduation of variation (Fig. 4.1 & 4.2) indicating that RPL37A would be the best choice as a normalizing gene for this project.

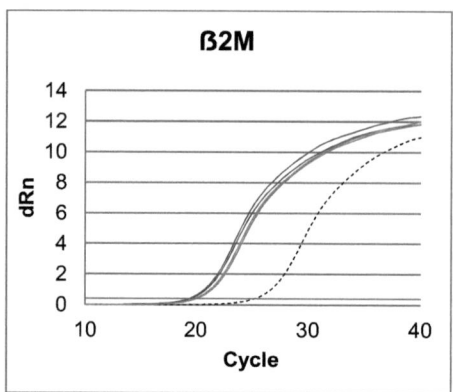

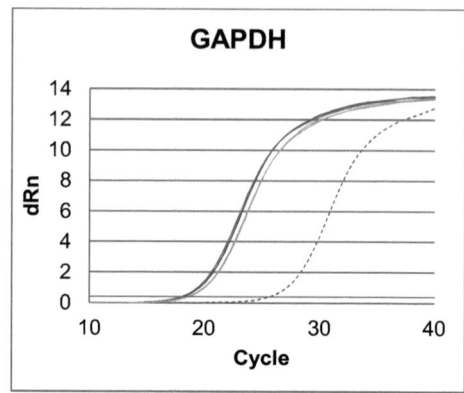

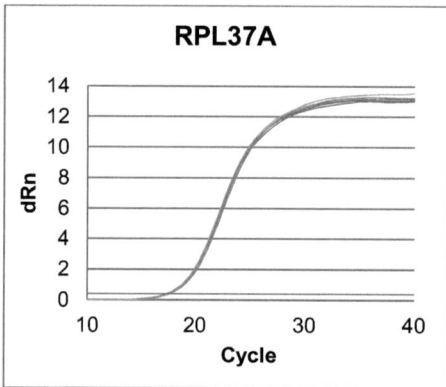

Fig. 4.1a-c Amplification curves of ß2M, GAPDH and RPL37A

These three charts visualize the robustness of the genes when treated with the toxin cocktail. The red horizontal line represents the threshold whilst the dashed lines represent the deviation.

ß2M shows some degree of variation and primer inefficiency whereas GAPDH has good primer efficiency but poor robustness. RPL37A shows good primer efficiency and good robustness against the treatment.

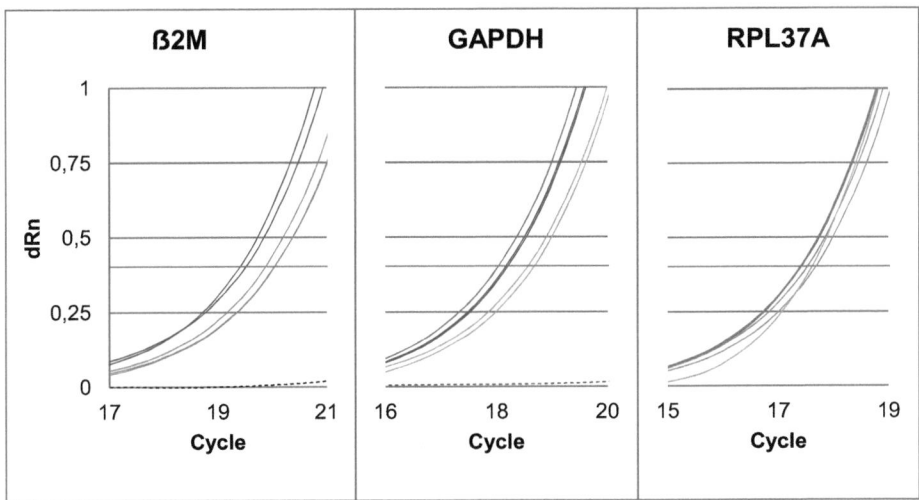

Fig. 4.2 Close-up on the region of threshold

This figure emphasizes the visually assessed robustness of RPL37A. The cycle range is 4 cycles

The statistical analysis of the Cts that were conducted using Medcalc, ultimately confirms the suitability of RPL37A as the reference gene. Due to the apparent inhibition in one of the samples, which caused errors in the ß2M and GAPDH reactions, the calculations of standard deviations and variations were performed without them and plotted together with statistical dataset properties on box-and-whisker plots.

Tab. 4.2 Statistical properties of the RG selection experiment

	N	Mean	Variance	SD	Median	Minimum	Maximum
w/ outliers							
ß2M	6	20,65	5,10	2,26	19,94	19,33	25,22
GAPDH	6	19,45	8,91	2,98	18,32	18,03	25,57
RPL37A	6	17,43	0,01	0,12	17,39	17,32	17,60
w/o outliers							
ß2M	5	19,74	0,11	0,34	19,84	19,33	20,04
GAPDH	5	18,28	0,06	0,25	18,16	18,03	18,60
RPL37A	6	17,43	0,01	0,12	17,39	17,32	17,60

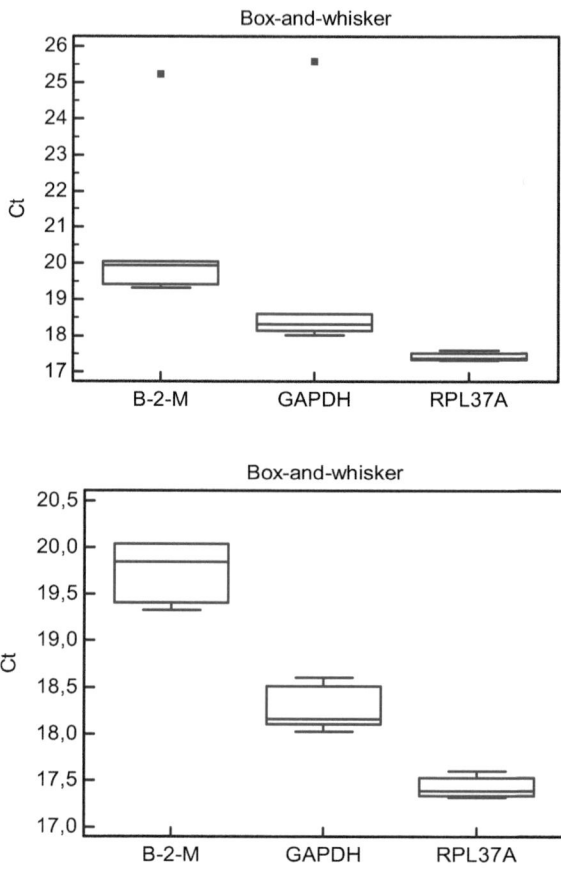

Fig. 4.3 Box-and-whisker plots of the Ct values with (top) and without outliers (bottom)

The aberrant Ct values are clearly outside the 3 SD range calculated without them. In the absence of the deviant Ct values, the variance of RPL37A is still significantly smaller than that of ß2M and GAPDH.

The subsequent melting curve analysis (Fig. 4.4) shows no detectable unspecific amplification or primer dimer formation.

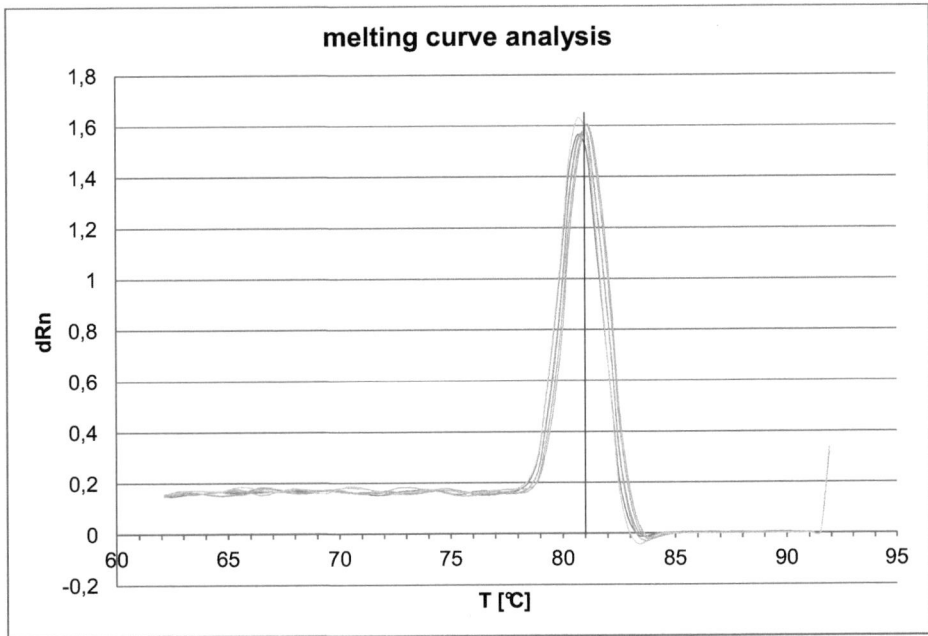

Fig. 4.4 Melting curves of RPL37A replicates

Regardless of toxin treatment, all replicate show similar melting points in the range around 81 ℃. Further, no significant amplification of unspecific products or dimeric products is detected.

4.1.2. Genes of interest

The adjustment of the optimal annealing temperature to 60 °C resulted in specific amplification of the cDNA template of the genes of interest (GOIs) as shown in Fig. 4.5.

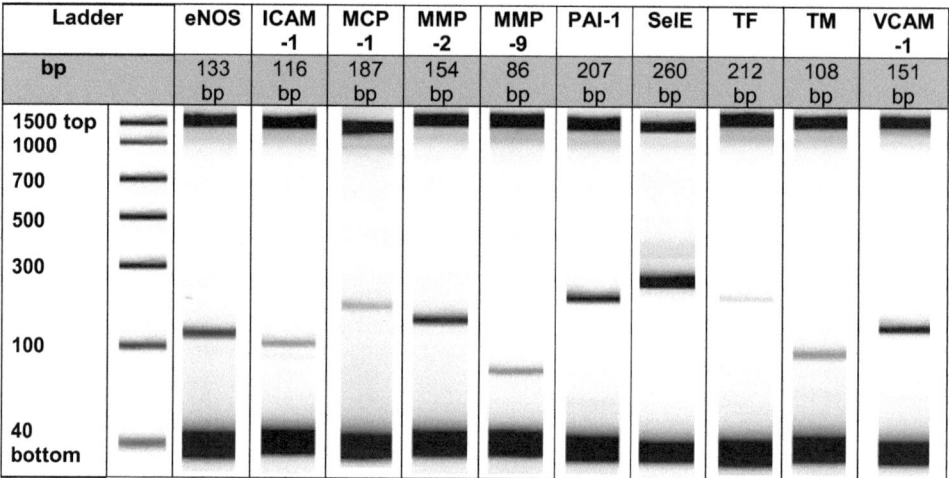

Ladder		eNOS	ICAM-1	MCP-1	MMP-2	MMP-9	PAI-1	SelE	TF	TM	VCAM-1
bp		133 bp	116 bp	187 bp	154 bp	86 bp	207 bp	260 bp	212 bp	108 bp	151 bp
1500 top 1000											
700											
500											
300											
100											
40 bottom											

Fig. 4.5 Overview of the GOI amplicons

All primers show specific amplification

The suitability of the primers for qPCR application was determined to be acceptable, even for those generating amplicons greater than the recommended 70-200 bp range (Bio-Rad Laboratories, 2006). To minimize the probability of mispriming to an undesired template and oligonucleotides, some primers had to be designed slightly larger. During the assessment of qPCR suitability, the amplicon melting temperatures (Tms, Tab. 4.3) have been determined to be over the Tms of the primers from negative template controls (ntc), if at all amplified (data not shown).

The relative primer efficiency testing (3.1.6.) was needed to compare the amplification of the GOIs and the RG. The satisfactory results are presented in Tab. 4.4 while Fig. 4.6 visualizes them.

Tab. 4.3 Numerical results of the relative primer efficiency assessment

Template [ng]	Ct						
	RPL37A(R)	eNOS(e)	TM(T)	VCAM(V)	ΔR_e	ΔR_T	ΔR_V
48,00	15,92	22,46	23,63	27,31	6,55	7,72	11,39
24,00	16,90	23,48	24,80	29,02	6,58	7,91	12,12
4,80	19,23	25,86	27,20	30,84	6,63	7,96	11,60
2,40	20,34	26,98	28,28	32,06	6,63	7,93	11,72
0,48	22,75	29,18	30,42	34,04	6,42	7,67	11,29
				mean:	6,56	7,84	11,62
				sdev:	0,08	0,13	0,32

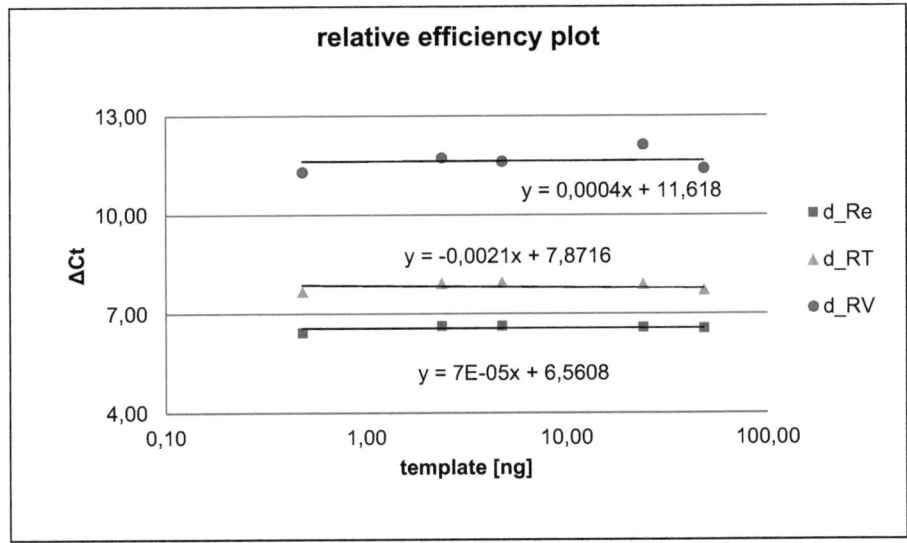

Fig. 4.6 Relative efficiency plot

This chart shows the primer efficiencies of eNOS (e), thrombomodulin (T) and VCAM-1 (V) relative to the primer efficiencies of RPL37A.

Due to the slope ranges being between -0,1 to 0,1, the primer efficiencies are to be considered comparable.

4.2.   Experiments

The following charts will visualize the expression behavior of the GOIs. In each chart, the lighter color represents experiment 1 (without E_2 treatment) while the darker color experiment 2 (with E_2 treatment). The data used for the visualization was constructed by applying the $2^{-\Delta\Delta Ct}$ method using the treated and untreated cells of each incubation time.

4.2.1. Endothelial nitric oxide synthase

As described earlier (Zhou et al., 2000), endotoxins down-regulate the expression of eNOS. The typical response to inflammatory/toxin stimulation is also demonstrated in the experiments performed (Fig. 4.7). Indoxyl sulfate might be the main reason for this result since it significantly reduces the expression of eNOS. Notably, in the cells with long term toxin treatment (24 h), eNOS seems to even surpass its initial level. Since eNOS has a negative feedback control regulation with NO, this might explain the late up-regulation.

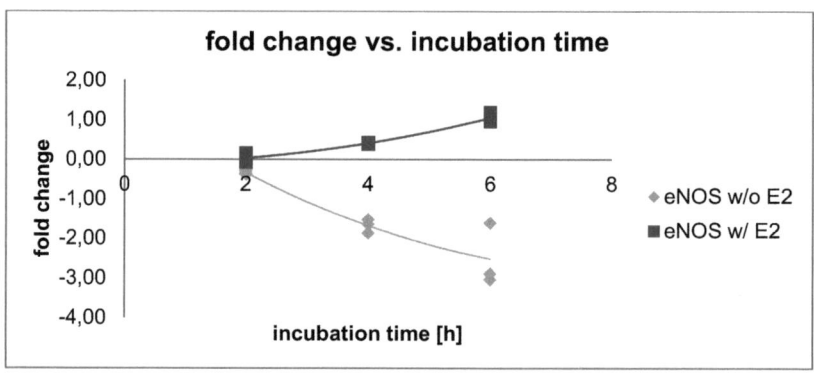

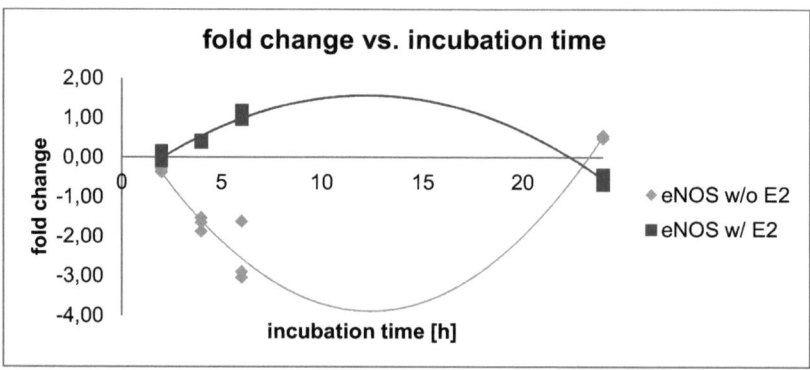

Fig. 4.7 eNOS expression charts

As opposed to the results without E_2 treatment, estrogen expectedly raises the eNOS level. This reaction is typical since a higher level of eNOS is also determined in premenopausal women. Hence, the assumption stands that eNOS has a protective effect on the cell which counteracts the inhibitory effect of indoxyl sulfate.

4.2.2. Intercellular adhesion molecule 1

Already at an early stage, ICAM-1 seems to be slightly up-regulated. Usually, the expression of ICAM-1 was shown to reach a high level after > 20 hours. In this case, it seems to have a reaction to an early stimulation either through some sort of stress or through interaction with the toxins. The unusual throwback to the initial level has yet to be investigated. Also, the possible diverse effects of individual or combined toxins at an early or late stage can be the cause of the negative parabolic expression curve depicted in the 24 h chart (Fig. 4.8). Estrogen reduces the expression as expected, supporting the cardioprotective effect of it (Piercy et al., 2002).

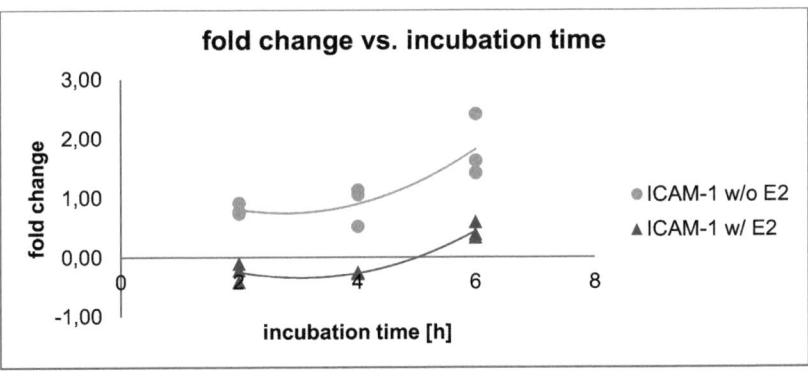

Fig. 4.8a ICAM-1 expression chart

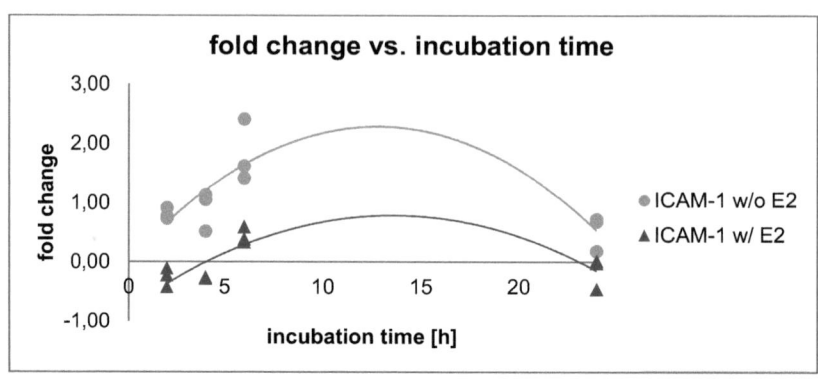

Fig. 4.8b ICAM-1 expression chart

4.2.3.   Monocyte chemotactic protein 1

The role of this cytokine in cardiovascular diseases is that it attracts other proteins and lipids to the inflammation site, hence resulting in an accelerated calcification of the vascular wall. Studies show that the up-regulation of MCP-1 is stimulated in diverse cells and by many factors such as endotoxins. The protein binding toxins cause a strong up-regulation of MCP-1 with the highest expression rate between 4 and 8 hours and a maximum between 12 and 20 hours. These values stand with the condition of valid 24 h values. Estrogen reduces the expression of MCP-1 on a strong level, which has already been discovered *in vivo* (mice) and *in vitro* (murine fibroblasts) (Fanti et al., 2003; Kovacs et al., 1996). While treatment without estrogen causes a drawback, the expression level after 24 hours is still at ~4 fold change while the fold change of the estrogen treated cells overall remains <1. The results of this expression analysis are highly comparable to the ones documented in literature, thus pointing to the strong anti-inflammatory effect of estrogen.

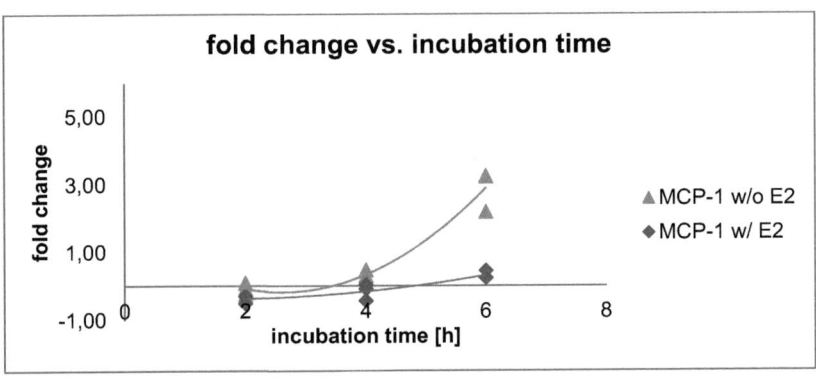

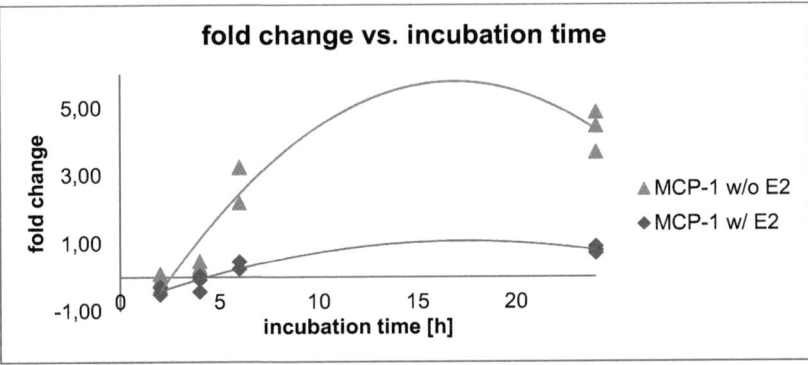

Fig. 4.9 MCP-1 expression charts

4.2.4. Matrix metalloprotease 2

Although literature reveals a negative regulation of MMP-2 by polyamines, this effect was scarcely observable in this experiment. A strong (positive) parabolic expression curve may yet again indicate either a more complex and timely differentiated interaction of the toxins on the expression of MMP-2 or an assay generated error causing it to have the beginning and the end of the curve around the same region well above the baseline, therefore indicating an upward shift of the curve. In the same range of ± 1 fold change, the estrogen treated cells show a negative parabolic expression curve that starts and ends around the baseline. The up-regulatory effect could be credited to the estrogen, since it has been documented to regulate MMP-2 expression in mammary tumor cells (Stabellini et al., 2005).

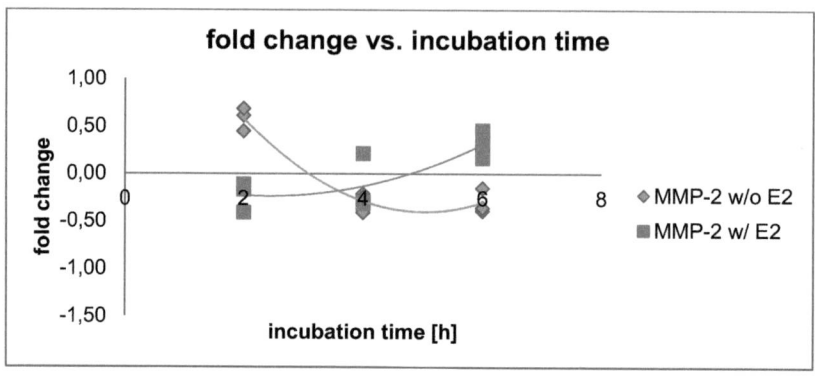

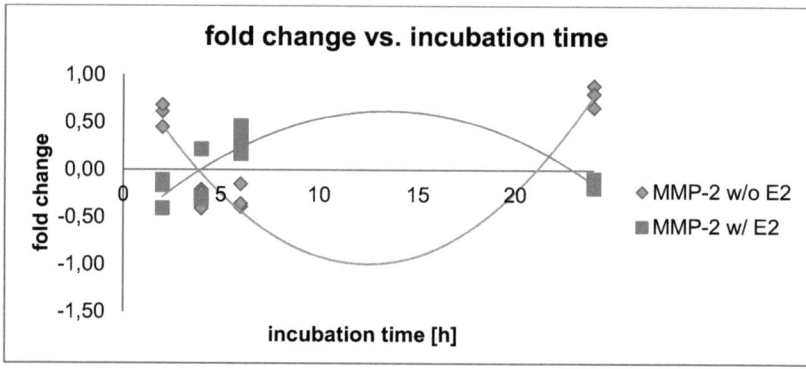

Fig. 4.10 MMP-2 expression charts

4.2.5. Matrix metalloprotease 9

Compared to MMP-2, MMP-9 shows a strong up-regulation after toxin stimulation. In addition, the overexpression of MMP-9 is linked to inflammation and post-myocardial infarct tissue remodeling. Due to the fact that advanced uremia has a high risk of causing a cardiovascular disease the inflammatory response to uremic toxin stimulation by up-regulating the MMP-9 expression is a very likely reaction (Halade, Jin, & Lindsey, 2013). Since it is an inflammatory response, the down-regulation of MMP-9 in estrogen treated cells also correlates with the anti-inflammatory effect of physiological estrogen.

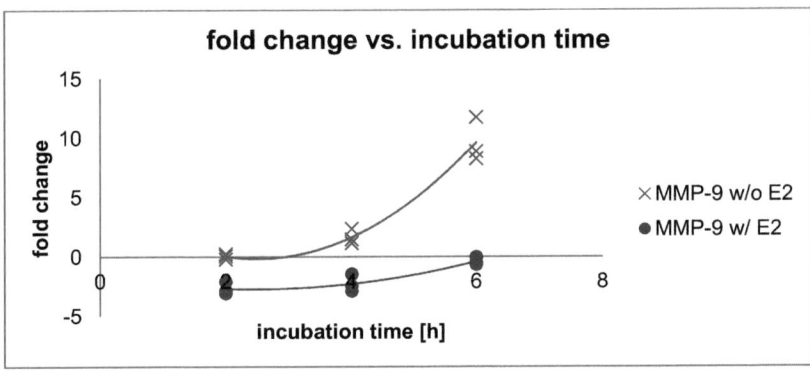

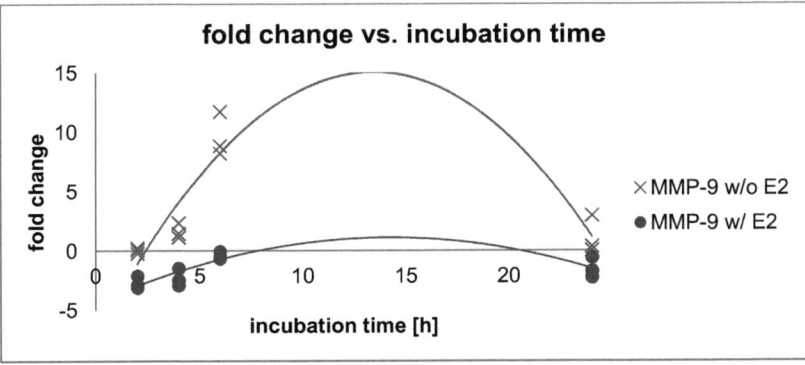

Fig. 4.11 MMP-9 expression charts

4.2.6.   Plasminogen activator inhibitor 1

Research has revealed that uremic toxins, especially indoxyl sulfate, cause the activation of NF-κB which in turn causes up-regulation of PAI-1 in HK-2 human renal proximal tubular cells (Motojima, Hosokawa, Yamato, Muraki, & Yoshioka, 2003). It seems that the same effect also occurs in HCAECs. Another analysis showed the up-regulation of PAI-1 in HUVECs by physiological estrogen concentrations in the medium. Said regulation involves the estrogen receptor α and cascade proteins such as G proteins, phosphatidylinositol-3-OH kinase, ρ-associated kinase II, c-Jun and c-Fos which in turn cause the up-regulation of estrogen induced PAI-1 (Gopal et al., 2012). Further, NF-κB has been proven to be activated by indoxyl sulfate in HUVECs (Tumur, Shimizu, Enomoto, Miyazaki, & Niwa, 2010). The data shows some upregulation of toxin treated cells as well as a reduced PAI-1 upregulation of estrogen treated cells compared to non-treated cells. More complex toxin interaction resulting in cell signaling dysfunction is also a possibility and could be the cause of the observed effect of uremic toxin and estrogen co-treatment of HCAECs.

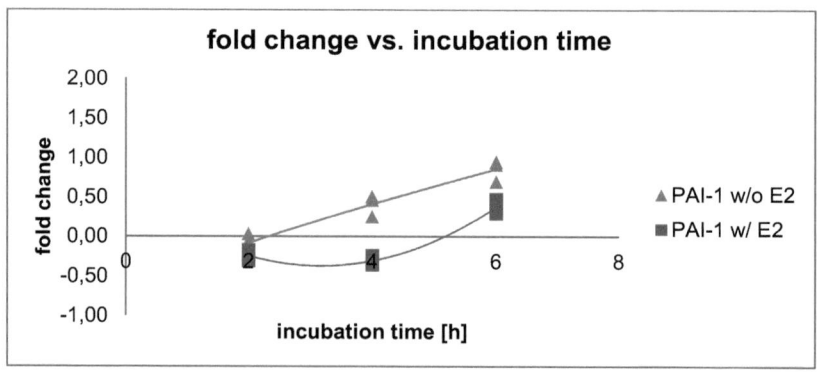

Fig. 4.12a PAI-1 expression chart

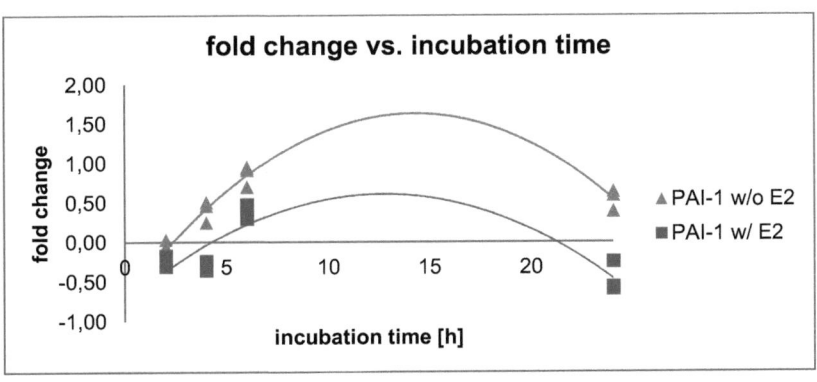

Fig. 4.12b PAI-1 expression chart

4.2.7.　E-selectin

According to previous publications (Leeuwenberg et al., 1992), the overexpression of E-selectin can be stimulated by cytokines and endotoxins, with a maximum reached after 6-12 hours and a final baseline concentration after ~ 24 hours measured by ELISA. Contrary to the study, E-selectin in this experiment is constantly being over-expressed and does not cease after 24 hours. The fold change values of the 4 hours incubation seem biased as biological expressions do not drop and rise in such a manner without corresponding environmental changes. A methodological error is likely responsible for these discordant results. Nevertheless, the upwards trend is still present. Since gene expression does not automatically result in functional protein secretion, a posttranscriptional regulation is highly probable, hence giving a possible explanation for the discrepancy between literature and the observed data. Other research has shown that indoxyl sulfate is responsible for E-selectin over-expression in HUVECs (Ito et al., 2010). A further *in vivo* experiment in rats revealed the reduced upregulation of E-selectin in female compared to male subjects when caused by an endotoxin-induced uveitis (Miyamoto et al., 1999). Ovarectomized female subjects also showed higher E-selectin expression. Estrogen treatment of male and ovarectomized female subjects reduced the E-selectin expression, hence coinciding with this experiment that shows a reduced upregulation of E-selectin that reaches a plateau after ~20 hours compared to cells without estrogen treatment.

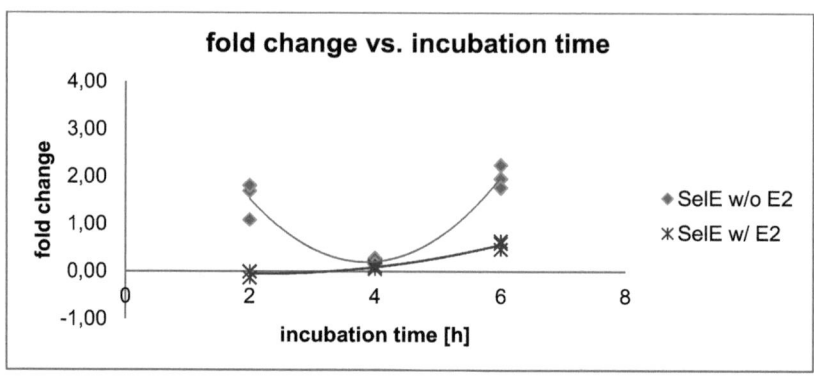

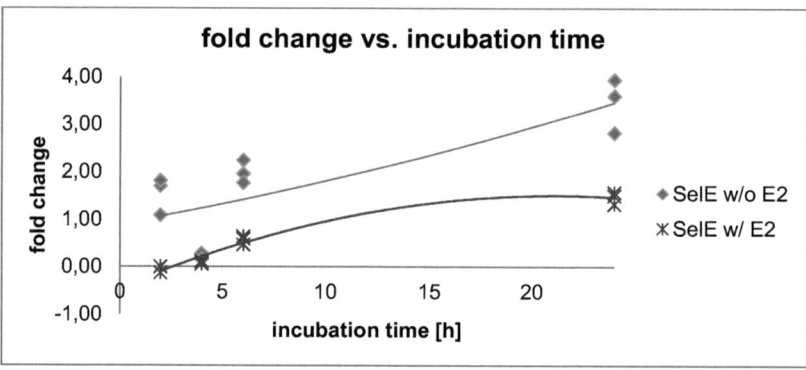

Fig. 4.13 E-selectin expression charts

4.2.8. Thrombomodulin

Seeing how a reduced Thrombomodulin level facilitates blood coagulation, negative regulation can be interpreted as a correlation between uremia and blood coagulation disorders in patients. Estrogen seems to counteract the toxins' regulatory effects. The biological significance of these findings is questionable since all fold changes are at a low level around the baseline.

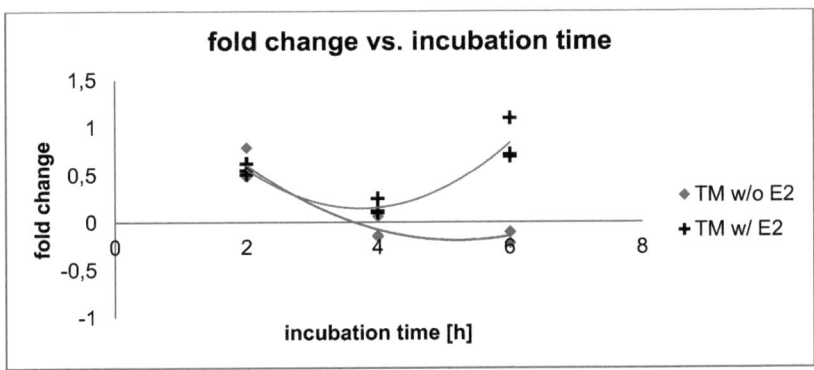

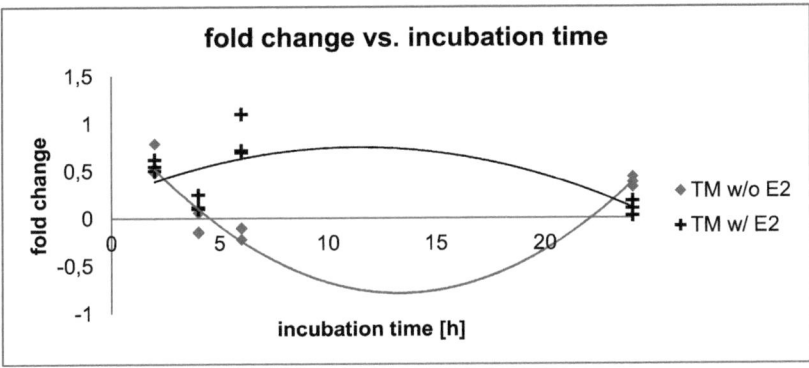

Fig. 4.14 TM expression charts

4.2.9. Tissue factor

Indoxyl sulfate most likely caused a highly positive fold change in the toxin treated cells (Gondouin et al., 2013). This finding is in alignment with the assumption that patients with chronic kidney disease also possess a blood coagulation disorder. Estrogen also seems to have a short upregulatory effect at the onset of treatment that returns to the baseline rather quickly, thus apparently antagonizing the effect of the toxins. Another possible interpretation of this finding is that there may be an initial lag in the pathways involved in estrogen/toxin-stimulated TF regulation, therefore causing a short peak with a subsequent down-regulation of Tissue Factor in estrogen treated cells.

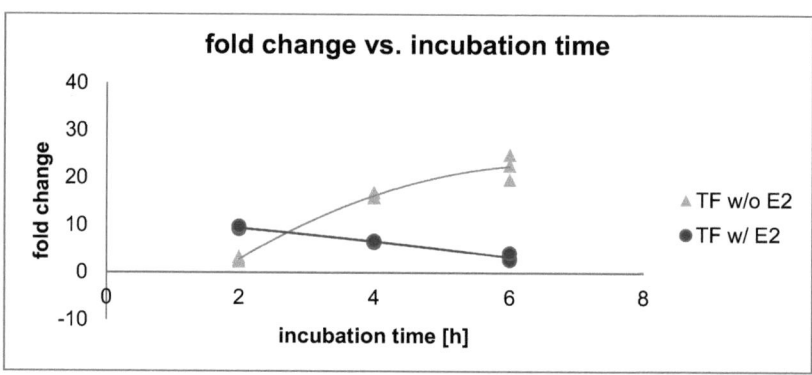

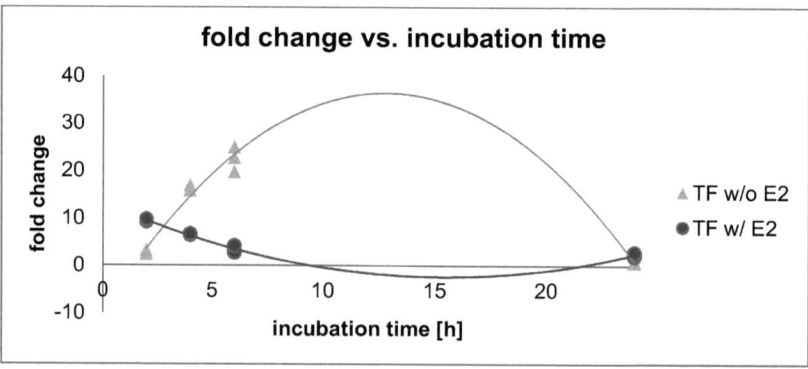

Fig. 4.15 TF expression charts

4.2.10.   Vascular cell adhesion molecule 1

Although some experiments have shown a down-regulatory effect of p-cresol on VCAM-1 expression in HUVECs (Dou et al., 2002), all toxins used in this experiment seem to cause an over-expression of VCAM-1. Given that uremia causes cardiovascular inflammation, the elevated levels are in alignment with the results of ICAM-1, and thus giving the results a high degree of validity. The anti-inflammatory properties of estrogen once again cause a significantly reduced VCAM-1 expression analogous to ICAM-1.

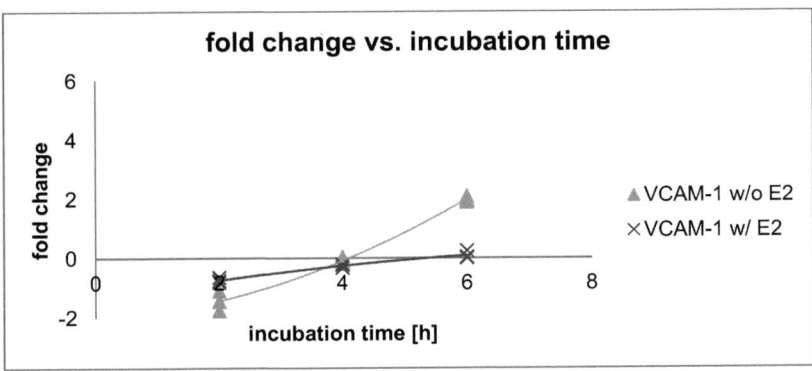

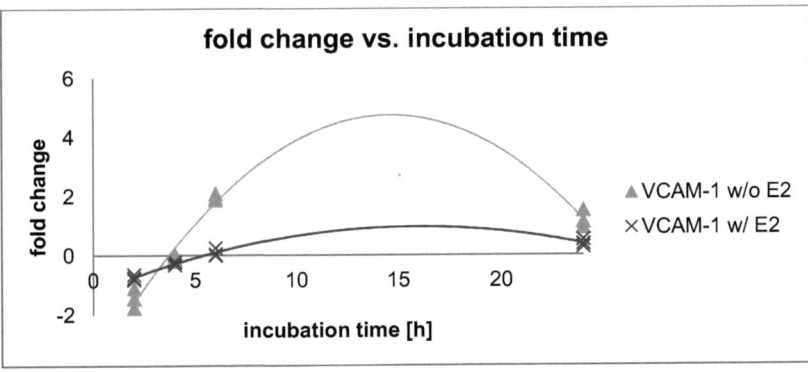

Fig. 4.16 VCAM-1 expression chart

5. Conclusion & Outlook

The majority of results obtained from these experiments support the knowledge that uremic toxins cause an over-expression of inflammatory parameters in HCAECs which facilitate wall-thickening and calcification of the vascular vessels as well as vascular tone dysfunction. The congruence of these results with the ones found in literature increases the relevance of this thesis. However, other parameters such as MMP-2 and E-selectin should be retested with similar or modified assay conditions to test for an assay-specific error or the presence of biological variability.

The influence of estrogen resulted in very compelling data. The statistics indicate a lower likelihood of cardiovascular disease morbidity in pre-menopausal women than in men and post-menopausal women. The results of this thesis highly support this indication since estrogen caused cardioprotective and anti-inflammatory results as well as a beneficial down-regulation of Tissue Factor.

Supplementary testing of inconclusive results including a proper protein analysis should be performed in futures trials in order to study the behavior of these proteins and their expression when stimulated with uremic toxins. Further, the long incubation responsiveness of the cells in the HBSS/HSA medium should be retested, since almost all genes showed atypical behavior after an incubation of 24 hours.

Abbreviations

CAD	coronary artery disease
cDNA	complementary DNA
CHD	coronary heart disease
CKD	chronic kidney disease
Ct	cycle of threshold
CVD	cardiovascular disease
dRn	delta Rn, magnitude of fluorescence in qPCR
E_2	17ß-estradiol
EMA	European Medicines Agency
eNOS	endothelial nitric oxide synthase
FDA	Food and Drug Administration
G6PDH	glucose-6-phosphate dehydrogenase
GAPDH	glyceraldehyd-3-phosphate dehydrogenase
gDNA	genomic DNA
GOI / POI	gene of interest / protein of interest
HBSS	Hanks' balanced salt solution
HCAEC	human coronary artery endothelial cell
HK-2	human renal proximal tubular cell
HSA	human serum albumin
HUVEC	human umbilical vein endothelial cell
HUWE1	E3 ubiquitin-protein ligase
ICAM-1	intercellular cell adhesion molecule 1
IL-1	interleukin 1
MCP-1	monocyte chemotactic protein 1
MMP-2/9	matrix metalloprotease 2/9
NF-κB	nuclear factor kappa B
NO	nitric oxide
PAI-1	plasminogen activator inhibitor 1

POLR2A	DNA-directed RNA polymerase II subunit RPB1
qPCR	quantitative real-time PCR
RG	reference gene
RPL37A	60S ribosomal protein L37a
SelE	endothelial selectin
ß2M	beta 2 microglobulin
TF	Tissue Factor
TGF-β	tumor growth factor beta
TM	Thrombomodulin
Tm	melting temperature of an amplicon
TNF-α	tumor necrosis factor alpha
VCAM-1	vascular cell adhesion molecule 1

References

Aoyama, I., Miyazaki, T., & Niwa, T. (1999). Preventive effects of an oral sorbent on nephropathy in rats. *Miner Electrolyte Metab, 25*(4-6), 365-372. doi: 57476

Arieff, A. I., & Massry, S. G. (1974). Calcium metabolism of brain in acute renal failure. Effects of uremia, hemodialysis, and parathyroid hormone. *J Clin Invest, 53*(2), 387-392. doi: 10.1172/JCI107571

Bio-Rad Laboratories, I., ,. (2006) Real-Time PCR Applications Guide.

Brunet, P., Dou, L., Cerini, C., & Berland, Y. (2003). Protein-bound uremic retention solutes. *Adv Ren Replace Ther, 10*(4), 310-320.

Burns, A. R., Takei, F., & Doerschuk, C. M. (1994). Quantitation of ICAM-1 expression in mouse lung during pneumonia. *J Immunol, 153*(7), 3189-3198.

Carr, M. W., Roth, S. J., Luther, E., Rose, S. S., & Springer, T. A. (1994). Monocyte chemoattractant protein 1 acts as a T-lymphocyte chemoattractant. *Proc Natl Acad Sci U S A, 91*(9), 3652-3656.

Castellino, F. J., & Ploplis, V. A. (2005). Structure and function of the plasminogen/plasmin system. *Thromb Haemost, 93*(4), 647-654. doi: 10.1267/THRO05040647

Centers for Disease Control and Prevention. (2012). Health, United States: U.S. Department of Health & Human Services.

Chakravorty, S. J., & Craig, A. (2005). The role of ICAM-1 in Plasmodium falciparum cytoadherence. *Eur J Cell Biol, 84*(1), 15-27. doi: 10.1016/j.ejcb.2004.09.002

Chen, Q., Zhang, X. H., & Massague, J. (2011). Macrophage binding to receptor VCAM-1 transmits survival signals in breast cancer cells that invade the lungs. *Cancer Cell, 20*(4), 538-549. doi: 10.1016/j.ccr.2011.08.025

Chen, V. M. (2013). Tissue factor de-encryption, thrombus formation, and thiol-disulfide exchange. *Semin Thromb Hemost, 39*(1), 40-47. doi: 10.1055/s-0032-1333311

Clarke, M. C., Littlewood, T. D., Figg, N., Maguire, J. J., Davenport, A. P., Goddard, M., & Bennett, M. R. (2008). Chronic apoptosis of vascular smooth muscle cells accelerates atherosclerosis and promotes calcification and medial degeneration. *Circ Res, 102*(12), 1529-1538. doi: 10.1161/CIRCRESAHA.108.175976

Collins, M. D., & East, A. K. (1998). Phylogeny and taxonomy of the food-borne pathogen Clostridium botulinum and its neurotoxins. *J Appl Microbiol, 84*(1), 5-17.

Colovic, Z., Pesutic-Pisac, V., Poljak, N. K., Racic, G., Cikojevic, D., & Kontic, M. (2013). Expression of matrix metalloproteinase-9 in patients with squamous cell carcinoma of the larynx. *Coll Antropol, 37*(1), 151-155.

De Smet, R., Van Kaer, J., Van Vlem, B., De Cubber, A., Brunet, P., Lameire, N., & Vanholder, R. (2003). Toxicity of free p-cresol: a prospective and cross-sectional analysis. *Clin Chem, 49*(3), 470-478.

Dolezalova, H., Stepita-Klauco, M., & Fairweather, R. (1974). An elevated cadaverine content in the brain of dormant mice. *Brain Res, 77*(1), 166-168.

Dou, L., Cerini, C., Brunet, P., Guilianelli, C., Moal, V., Grau, G., . . . Berland, Y. (2002). P-cresol, a uremic toxin, decreases endothelial cell response to inflammatory cytokines. *Kidney Int, 62*(6), 1999-2009. doi: 10.1046/j.1523-1755.2002.t01-1-00651.x

Egelund, R., Rodenburg, K. W., Andreasen, P. A., Rasmussen, M. S., Guldberg, R. E., & Petersen, T. E. (1998). An ester bond linking a fragment of a serine proteinase to its serpin inhibitor. *Biochemistry, 37*(18), 6375-6379. doi: 10.1021/bi973043+

European Medicines Agency. (2012). European Medicines Agency decision reports: European Medicines Agency.

Fanti, P., Nazareth, M., Bucelli, R., Mineo, M., Gibbs, K., Kumin, M., . . . Aronica, S. M. (2003). Estrogen decreases chemokine levels in murine mammary tissue: implications for the regulatory role of MIP-1 alpha and MCP-1/JE in mammary tumor formation. *Endocrine, 22*(2), 161-168.

Food and Drug Administration. (2013). Press Announcements 2013. Retrieved 26. Jul., 2013, from http://www.fda.gov/newsevents/newsroom/PressAnnouncements/ default.htm

Gallicchio, M., Argyriou, S., Ianches, G., Filonzi, E. L., Zoellner, H., Hamilton, J. A., . . . Wojta, J. (1994). Stimulation of PAI-1 expression in endothelial cells by cultured vascular smooth muscle cells. *Arterioscler Thromb, 14*(5), 815-823.

Gondouin, B., Cerini, C., Dou, L., Sallee, M., Duval-Sabatier, A., Pletinck, A., . . . Burtey, S. (2013). Indolic uremic solutes increase tissue factor production in endothelial cells by the aryl hydrocarbon receptor pathway. *Kidney Int, 84*(4), 733-744. doi: 10.1038/ki.2013.133

Gopal, S., Garibaldi, S., Goglia, L., Polak, K., Palla, G., Spina, S., . . . Simoncini, T. (2012). Estrogen regulates endothelial migration via plasminogen activator inhibitor (PAI-1). *Mol Hum Reprod, 18*(8), 410-416. doi: 10.1093/molehr/gas011

Greve, J. M., Davis, G., Meyer, A. M., Forte, C. P., Yost, S. C., Marlor, C. W., . . . McClelland, A. (1989). The major human rhinovirus receptor is ICAM-1. *Cell, 56*(5), 839-847.

Griscavage, J. M., Hobbs, A. J., & Ignarro, L. J. (1995). Negative modulation of nitric oxide synthase by nitric oxide and nitroso compounds. *Adv Pharmacol, 34*, 215-234.

Halade, G. V., Jin, Y. F., & Lindsey, M. L. (2013). Matrix metalloproteinase (MMP)-9: a proximal biomarker for cardiac remodeling and a distal biomarker for inflammation. *Pharmacol Ther, 139*(1), 32-40. doi: 10.1016/j.pharmthera.2013.03.009

Hermann, M., Seif, F., Schneider, W. J., & Ivessa, N. E. (1997). Estrogen dependence of synthesis and secretion of apolipoprotein B-containing lipoproteins in the chicken hepatoma cell line, LMH-2A. *J Lipid Res, 38*(7), 1308-1317.

Hopkins, A. M., Baird, A. W., & Nusrat, A. (2004). ICAM-1: targeted docking for exogenous as well as endogenous ligands. *Adv Drug Deliv Rev, 56*(6), 763-778. doi: 10.1016/j.addr.2003.10.043

Hu, J., Mahmoud, M. I., & el-Fakahany, E. E. (1994). Polyamines inhibit nitric oxide synthase in rat cerebellum. *Neurosci Lett, 175*(1-2), 41-45.

Ito, S., Osaka, M., Higuchi, Y., Nishijima, F., Ishii, H., & Yoshida, M. (2010). Indoxyl sulfate induces leukocyte-endothelial interactions through up-regulation of E-selectin. *J Biol Chem, 285*(50), 38869-38875. doi: 10.1074/jbc.M110.166686

Jankowski, J., Luftmann, H., Tepel, M., Leibfritz, D., Zidek, W., & Schluter, H. (1998). Characterization of dimethylguanosine, phenylethylamine, and phenylacetic acid as inhibitors of Ca2+ ATPase in end-stage renal failure. *J Am Soc Nephrol, 9*(7), 1249-1257.

Jankowski, J., van der Giet, M., Jankowski, V., Schmidt, S., Hemeier, M., Mahn, B., . . . Tepel, M. (2003). Increased plasma phenylacetic acid in patients with end-stage renal failure inhibits iNOS expression. *J Clin Invest, 112*(2), 256-264. doi: 10.1172/JCI15524

Jourde-Chiche, N., Dou, L., Cerini, C., Dignat-George, F., & Brunet, P. (2011). Vascular incompetence in dialysis patients--protein-bound uremic toxins and endothelial dysfunction. *Semin Dial, 24*(3), 327-337. doi: 10.1111/j.1525-139X.2011.00925.x

Jousilahti, P., Vartiainen, E., Tuomilehto, J., & Puska, P. (1999). Sex, age, cardiovascular risk factors, and coronary heart disease: a prospective follow-up study of 14 786 middle-aged men and women in Finland. *Circulation, 99*(9), 1165-1172.

Konigsberg, W., Kirchhofer, D., Riederer, M. A., & Nemerson, Y. (2001). The TF:VIIa complex: clinical significance, structure-function relationships and its role in signaling and metastasis. *Thromb Haemost, 86*(3), 757-771.

Kovacs, E. J., Faunce, D. E., Ramer-Quinn, D. S., Mott, F. J., Dy, P. W., & Frazier-Jessen, M. R. (1996). Estrogen regulation of JE/MCP-1 mRNA expression in fibroblasts. *J Leukoc Biol, 59*(4), 562-568.

Leeuwenberg, J. F., Smeets, E. F., Neefjes, J. J., Shaffer, M. A., Cinek, T., Jeunhomme, T. M., . . . Buurman, W. A. (1992). E-selectin and intercellular adhesion molecule-1 are released by activated human endothelial cells in vitro. *Immunology, 77*(4), 543-549.

Liu, J., Hughes, T. E., & Sessa, W. C. (1997). The first 35 amino acids and fatty acylation sites determine the molecular targeting of endothelial nitric oxide synthase into the Golgi region of cells: a green fluorescent protein study. *J Cell Biol, 137*(7), 1525-1535.

Livak, K. J., & Schmittgen, T. D. (2001). Analysis of relative gene expression data using real-time quantitative PCR and the 2(-Delta Delta C(T)) Method. *Methods, 25*(4), 402-408. doi: 10.1006/meth.2001.1262

Mackay, J., Mensah, G. A., Mendis, S., Greenlund, K., & World Health Organization. (2004). *The atlas of heart disease and stroke.* Geneva: World Health Organization.

Maltseva, D. V., Khaustova, N. A., Fedotov, N. N., Matveeva, E. O., Lebedev, A. E., Shkurnikov, M. U., . . . Tonevitsky, A. G. (2013). High-throughput identification of reference genes for research and clinical RT-qPCR analysis of breast cancer samples. *J Clin Bioinforma, 3*(1), 13. doi: 10.1186/2043-9113-3-13

Miyamoto, N., Mandai, M., Suzuma, I., Suzuma, K., Kobayashi, K., & Honda, Y. (1999). Estrogen protects against cellular infiltration by reducing the expressions of E-selectin and IL-6 in endotoxin-induced uveitis. *J Immunol, 163*(1), 374-379.

Motojima, M., Hosokawa, A., Yamato, H., Muraki, T., & Yoshioka, T. (2003). Uremic toxins of organic anions up-regulate PAI-1 expression by induction of NF-kappaB and free radical in proximal tubular cells. *Kidney Int, 63*(5), 1671-1680. doi: 10.1046/j.1523-1755.2003.00906.x

National Institutes of Health. (2013). Estimates of Funding for Various Research, Condition, and Disease Categories (RCDC). Retrieved 26. Jul., 2013, from http://report.nih.gov/categorical_spending.aspx

National Institutes of Health, & National Library of Medicines. (2011, 20. Jan.). Hazardous Substances Data Bank. Retrieved 14. Sept., 2013, from http://toxnet.nlm.nih.gov/cgi-bin/sis/htmlgen?HSDB

Niwa, T. (2010). Indoxyl sulfate is a nephro-vascular toxin. *J Ren Nutr, 20*(5 Suppl), S2-6. doi: 10.1053/j.jrn.2010.05.002

Niwa, T., & Shimizu, H. (2012). Indoxyl sulfate induces nephrovascular senescence. *J Ren Nutr, 22*(1), 102-106. doi: 10.1053/j.jrn.2011.10.032

Pero, R. W. (2010). Health consequences of catabolic synthesis of hippuric acid in humans. *Curr Clin Pharmacol, 5*(1), 67-73.

Piercy, K. T., Donnell, R. L., Kirkpatrick, S. S., Timaran, C. H., Stevens, S. L., Freeman, M. B., & Goldman, M. H. (2002). Effects of estrogen, progesterone, and combination exposure on interleukin-1 beta-induced expression of VCAM-1, ICAM-1, PECAM, and E-selectin by human female iliac artery endothelial cells. *J Surg Res, 105*(2), 215-219.

Piroddi, M., Bartolini, D., Ciffolilli, S., & Galli, F. (2013). Nondialyzable uremic toxins. *Blood Purif, 35 Suppl 2*, 30-41. doi: 10.1159/000350846

Raz, R., Chazan, B., & Dan, M. (2004). Cranberry juice and urinary tract infection. *Clin Infect Dis, 38*(10), 1413-1419. doi: 10.1086/386328

Roman, L. J., Martasek, P., Miller, R. T., Harris, D. E., de La Garza, M. A., Shea, T. M., . . . Masters, B. S. (2000). The C termini of constitutive nitric-oxide synthases control electron flow through the flavin and heme domains and affect modulation by calmodulin. *J Biol Chem, 275*(38), 29225-29232. doi: 10.1074/jbc.M004766200

Sarnak, M. J., Levey, A. S., Schoolwerth, A. C., Coresh, J., Culleton, B., Hamm, L. L., . . . Prevention. (2003). Kidney disease as a risk factor for development of cardiovascular disease: a statement from the American Heart Association Councils on Kidney in Cardiovascular Disease, High Blood Pressure Research, Clinical Cardiology, and Epidemiology and Prevention. *Circulation, 108*(17), 2154-2169. doi: 10.1161/01.CIR.0000095676.90936.80

Sharma, A. K., & Khanna, D. (2013). Diabetes mellitus associated cardiovascular signalling alteration: a need for the revisit. *Cell Signal, 25*(5), 1149-1155. doi: 10.1016/j.cellsig.2013.01.022

Stabellini, G., Moscheni, C., Gagliano, N., Dellavia, C., Calastrini, C., Ferioli, M. E., & Gioia, M. (2005). Depletion of polyamines and increase of transforming growth factor-beta1, c-myc, collagen-type I, matrix metalloproteinase-1, and metalloproteinase-2 mRNA in primary human gingival fibroblasts. *J Periodontol, 76*(3), 443-449. doi: 10.1902/jop.2005.76.3.443

The European Bioinformatics Institute. (2012, 03. Jul.). The database and ontology of Chemical Entities of Biological Interest. Retrieved 14. Nov., 2013, from http://www.ebi.ac.uk/chebi/

Thermo Fisher Scientific Inc. (2013). DNase I, RNase-free - Supporting Data. Retrieved 26. Jul., 2013, from http://www.thermoscientificbio.com/dna-and-rna-modifying-enzymes/dnase-i-rnase-free/

Til, H. P., Falke, H. E., Prinsen, M. K., & Willems, M. I. (1997). Acute and subacute toxicity of tyramine, spermidine, spermine, putrescine and cadaverine in rats. *Food Chem Toxicol, 35*(3-4), 337-348.

Tumur, Z., Shimizu, H., Enomoto, A., Miyazaki, H., & Niwa, T. (2010). Indoxyl sulfate upregulates expression of ICAM-1 and MCP-1 by oxidative stress-induced NF-kappaB activation. *Am J Nephrol, 31*(5), 435-441. doi: 10.1159/000299798

Verhagen, H. J., Heijnen-Snyder, G. J., Pronk, A., Vroom, T. M., van Vroonhoven, T. J., Eikelboom, B. C., . . . de Groot, P. G. (1996). Thrombomodulin activity on mesothelial cells: perspectives for mesothelial cells as an alternative for endothelial cells for cell seeding on vascular grafts. *Br J Haematol, 95*(3), 542-549.

Wagner, D. D. (1993). The Weibel-Palade body: the storage granule for von Willebrand factor and P-selectin. *Thromb Haemost, 70*(1), 105-110.

Waisman, D. M. (2003). *Plasminogen : structure, activation, and regulation.* New York: Kluwer Academic/Plenum Publishers.

World Health Organization. (2008). Health statistics and health information systems, Deaths estimates for 2008 by cause for WHO Member States. Retrieved 8. Nov., 2013, from http://www.who.int/healthinfo/global_burden_disease/estimates_country /en/

Yamamoto, K., Takeshita, K., Kojima, T., Takamatsu, J., & Saito, H. (2005). Aging and plasminogen activator inhibitor-1 (PAI-1) regulation: implication in the pathogenesis of thrombotic disorders in the elderly. *Cardiovasc Res, 66*(2), 276-285. doi: 10.1016/j.cardiores.2004.11.013

Yoshida, K., Yoneda, T., Kimura, S., Fujimoto, K., Okajima, E., & Hirao, Y. (2006). Polyamines as an inhibitor on erythropoiesis of hemodialysis patients by in vitro bioassay using the fetal mouse liver assay. *Ther Apher Dial, 10*(3), 267-272. doi: 10.1111/j.1744-9987.2006.00370.x

Zhou, X. J., Laszik, Z., Ni, Z., Wang, X. Q., Brackett, D. J., Lerner, M. R., . . . Vaziri, N. D. (2000). Down-regulation of renal endothelial nitric oxide synthase expression in experimental glomerular thrombotic microangiopathy. *Lab Invest, 80*(7), 1079-1087.

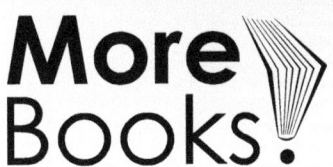
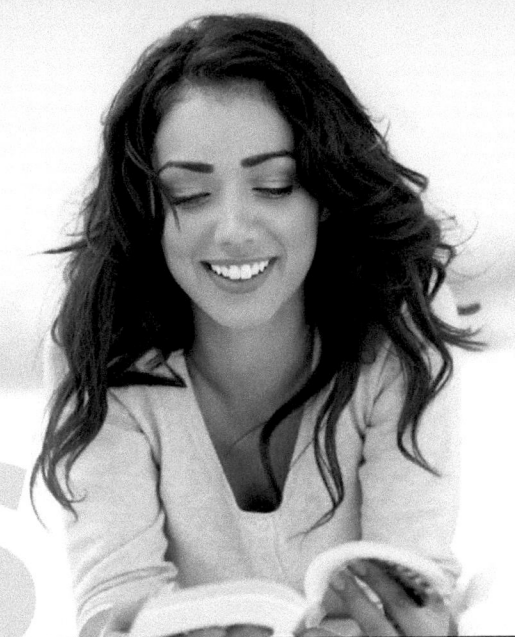

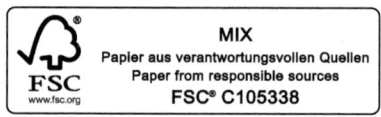